THRIVING BEYOND

SEIZURES

A Holistic Approach to Epilepsy Management, Offering Empowering Strategies and Practical Tools for Living a Life of Abundance

BY KARI WALLIS

Copyright © 2023 by Kari Wallis

About the Author

Dr. Kari Wallis, a distinguished neurologist, is committed to advancing the understanding and treatment of epilepsy. Having extensive knowledge and experience in the field, she brings a compassionate and comprehensive approach to patient care.

Renowned in neurological research, Dr. Wallis has significantly contributed to the development of innovative diagnostic procedures and therapeutic modalities for epilepsy. Her dedication to improving the quality of life for individuals affected by epilepsy is evident in both her clinical practice and academic pursuits.

Dr. Wallis embarked on her neurology journey driven by a passion for unraveling the complexities of the brain. Holding advanced degrees in neurology and neurophysiology, she has gained recognition for her groundbreaking work in diagnosing and managing epilepsy.

Beyond her clinical work, Dr. Wallis is a passionate advocate for epilepsy awareness and education. Through public lectures, community outreach programs, and collaborations with advocacy groups, she strives to dispel myths, reduce stigma, and create a supportive environment for individuals living with epilepsy.

"Thriving Beyond Seizures" stands as a testament to Dr. Wallis's commitment to providing valuable insights, empowering individuals, and fostering a sense of community within the epilepsy landscape. Her unwavering dedication to neurological care continues to have a profound impact on the lives of those touched by epilepsy.

Table of Contents

Introduction

Welcome to an immersive exploration into the intricate and nuanced world of epilepsy—a journey that transcends the clinical gaze to delve deeply into the human experience. In my capacity as a neurologist, I've been granted the privilege of witnessing the indomitable spirit of individuals navigating the complex terrain of neurological conditions. Yet, within this vast landscape, epilepsy emerges as a singular narrative, weaving itself intricately into the very fabric of life.

At the core of this guide lies a profound and multifaceted purpose—to stand as a beacon of understanding, empathy, and empowerment for those navigating the labyrinthine challenges of epilepsy. This book aspires to be more than a mere compendium of medical insights; it seeks to be a holistic companion, offering a comprehensive roadmap of strategies, perspectives, and a reservoir of collective wisdom aimed at enhancing the quality of life for individuals and their families living with epilepsy.

The purpose transcends mere information dissemination; it is a call to empower, guide, and inspire readers toward a life that transcends the limitations imposed by seizures. Allow me to invite you into the intimate corridors of my experience as a neurologist, where the mosaic of patient narratives forms the rich tapestry of understanding the human side of epilepsy. Among these stories, Sophia's journey stands out as a vivid testament to the complexities that extend far beyond a clinical diagnosis.

Beyond the confines of medical consultations, I delved into Sophia's dreams, aspirations, and the intricate tapestry of daily triumphs and tribulations woven into her life. Her story became a profound illumination, shedding light on the limitations of a purely clinical approach. It prompted a poignant realization—that thriving beyond seizures necessitates a deep acknowledgment of the person behind the diagnosis. In every heartbeat, Sophia's narrative underscores the deeply personal aspect of epilepsy—the dreams, struggles, and victories that collectively shape each individual's unique journey.

Regrettably, epilepsy carries not only the burden of neurological disruptions but also the weight of societal misconceptions and stigma. Dispelling seizures becomes more than a clinical endeavor; it transforms into a mission to challenge prejudice and foster a society that comprehends the nuanced challenges faced by individuals with epilepsy.

In Sophia's courageous journey, her resilience became a powerful retort to societal judgment. Her unwavering determination to confront this stigma emerged not merely as a personal triumph but as a beacon of hope and inspiration for others navigating the labyrinth of epilepsy. As we traverse the chapters that follow, our aim extends beyond challenging stereotypes; we aspire to nurture empathy and ignite open conversations that dismantle the walls of societal prejudice surrounding epilepsy.

The impact of epilepsy transcends the conventional boundaries of medical discourse. The holistic approach advocated in these pages is a clarion call to recognize that thriving beyond seizures is a multidimensional journey. It encompasses not only medical interventions but also extends its embrace to lifestyle adjustments, emotional well-being, and the invaluable support of a community. To thrive, in its truest sense, is to grasp the intricate interplay of these dimensions, acknowledging their collective influence on the holistic well-being of individuals with epilepsy.

Sophia's narrative, a mosaic painted with diverse experiences, revealed the multidimensional nature of epilepsy. While medical interventions remain pivotal, they represent just one facet of this intricate journey. Thriving involves navigating relationships, managing emotional well-being, advocating for one's rights, and crafting a lifestyle that not only accommodates but supports overall health and fulfillment.

As we turn the pages in the chapters that follow, each becomes a canvas—a canvas painted with the collective wisdom drawn from the amalgamation of clinical expertise and personal narratives. Together, let's embark on this expansive and immersive journey of understanding, growth, and empowerment. The goal surpasses the mere management of epilepsy; it is a collective endeavor to live abundantly despite the challenges and to thrive in the truest sense of the word.

In traversing this narrative landscape, remember, that you are not alone. The stories within these pages, whether from the perspective of a neurologist or the lived experiences of individuals, converge to form a tapestry of understanding, resilience, and shared humanity. The journey begins here, and I extend an invitation for you to fully immerse yourself in the chapters that follow as we collectively navigate life with epilepsy.

Chapter One: Understanding Epilepsy

In this chapter, we delve into the diverse spectrum of this neurological condition. Epilepsy encompasses unpredictable seizures, varying from subtle episodes to pronounced convulsions, significantly impacting individuals' lives. We explore different types and their distinguishing traits, highlighting the complexity beyond general perceptions. Unraveling potential triggers and causes, we navigate the multifaceted origins of seizures. Addressing societal attitudes and misconceptions, we aim to dispel myths and foster empathy within our communities. This foundational guide aims to enhance awareness and comprehension of epilepsy in its varied forms.

Definition and Overview

Epilepsy is a complex neurological disorder characterized by recurrent and unpredictable seizures. These seizures arise from abnormal electrical activity within the brain, creating a temporary disruption in the communication between nerve cells. The manifestations of epilepsy are vast and varied, spanning from subtle sensory disturbances such as peculiar smells or tastes to more pronounced convulsions and loss of consciousness. This intricate spectrum of symptoms highlights the heterogeneity of the condition, underlining the unique challenges faced by individuals grappling with epilepsy.

Beyond the immediate physical expressions of seizures, the impact of epilepsy permeates multiple facets of individuals' lives. The unpredictability of seizures introduces a pervasive element of uncertainty, affecting various daily activities. For instance, individuals with epilepsy may encounter restrictions on driving, impacting personal mobility and independence. Certain occupations may also be limited, contributing to challenges in career choices and financial stability.

The cumulative effect of these limitations can lead to a complex web of emotional and psychological consequences. Living with epilepsy often entails navigating a landscape of anxiety, depression, and a heightened sense of vulnerability. The stigma associated with seizures can foster social isolation, influencing relationships and the broader community's understanding of the condition.

The educational and employment spheres may be adversely affected, influencing self-esteem and overall quality of life. Recognizing the impact of epilepsy necessitates a holistic approach—one that goes beyond the surface-level manifestations of seizures to address the intricate interplay of biological, psychological, and social factors.

By delving into the multifaceted nature of epilepsy, we aim to cultivate a deeper understanding that transcends clinical descriptions. Through this understanding, we can foster empathy, dispel misconceptions, and pave the way for a more inclusive and supportive environment for individuals navigating the challenges posed by epilepsy.

Types and Variations

Epilepsy, manifests in a diverse array of types, each characterized by unique features that intricately shape the nature and presentation of seizures. A thorough exploration of these variations is pivotal for an accurate diagnosis, the formulation of personalized treatment plans, and the provision of nuanced support. Let's embark on a comprehensive journey through the major types of epilepsy, unraveling their distinguishing characteristics in intricate detail:

Focal (Partial) Epilepsy

Simple Partial Seizures: Simple partial seizures originate in a specific area of the brain and are marked by localized symptoms that do not affect consciousness. The manifestations are manifold, ranging from sensory changes such as tingling or strange smells to motor symptoms like twitching or involuntary movements. The specificity of these symptoms is contingent upon the precise region of the brain involved, adding a layer of complexity to their diagnosis and understanding.

Complex Partial Seizures: Complex partial seizures, on the other hand, impact consciousness and behavior. Often emanating from the temporal lobe, these seizures may involve auras, altered perceptions, and automatisms—repetitive, purposeless movements such as lip-smacking or hand-wringing. The intricate interplay of neural circuits during complex partial seizures contributes to the diversity of experiences reported by individuals.

Generalized Epilepsy

Absence Seizures: Commonly observed in childhood, absence seizures are characterized by brief lapses in consciousness. During these episodes, individuals may experience staring spells, eye blinking, or subtle movements. The rapid onset and offset of altered awareness make the diagnosis challenging, and a comprehensive understanding of the distinctive features is crucial for accurate recognition.

Tonic-Clonic Seizures: Tonic-clonic seizures, perhaps the most recognized type, exhibit distinct phases. The tonic phase involves muscle stiffness, often causing falls, while the clonic phase is marked by rhythmic jerking movements. Loss of consciousness, altered breathing patterns, and potential postictal confusion contribute to the complexity of these seizures.

Myoclonic Seizures: Myoclonic seizures present as sudden, brief jerking movements affecting various muscle groups. These movements can be subtle or severe, significantly impacting daily activities. Myoclonic seizures may occur in isolation or as part of broader epilepsy syndromes, emphasizing the intricate nature of their clinical presentation.

Atonic Seizures: Atonic seizures result in a sudden loss of muscle tone, leading to the person collapsing or falling. Often referred to as "drop attacks," these seizures pose a distinct risk of injury due to the abrupt loss of postural control. Understanding the dynamics of atonic seizures is crucial for implementing preventive measures.

Unique Seizure Types

Epileptic Spasms: Epileptic spasms are distinctive, and frequently observed in infancy. These seizures involve brief, repetitive muscle contractions, presenting as sudden bending forward or stiffening. Recognizing the specific features of epileptic spasms is essential for diagnosing underlying epilepsy syndromes, such as West syndrome.

Status Epilepticus: Status epilepticus represents a medical emergency, characterized by prolonged and continuous seizure activity without recovery between episodes. Immediate intervention is crucial to prevent potential complications, necessitating a profound understanding of the dynamic neurobiological processes involved.

Developmental Aspects

Epilepsy's impact extends beyond the immediate seizures, evolving over the lifespan. Understanding these developmental trajectories is paramount for tailoring effective treatment plans. For example, childhood absence epilepsy may transition into other generalized epilepsy syndromes during adolescence, such as juvenile myoclonic epilepsy, highlighting the necessity of a dynamic and evolving approach to care.

Cognitive and Psychiatric Comorbidities

Beyond seizures, epilepsy often coexists with cognitive and psychiatric challenges, adding layers of complexity to the clinical picture. Memory difficulties, mood disorders such as depression or anxiety, and attention deficits are common. Recognizing and addressing these additional dimensions is integral to providing comprehensive epilepsy care, as they profoundly influence an individual's overall well-being and quality of life.

In unraveling the diverse and intricate landscape of epilepsy, we gain profound insights into the multifaceted nature of this condition. This detailed understanding not only aids healthcare professionals in accurate diagnosis and effective treatment planning but also fosters a compassionate and informed approach to supporting individuals living with epilepsy through their unique and dynamic journey.

Etiology and Triggers

Epileptic seizures, characterized by abnormal electrical activity in the brain, are influenced by a complex interplay of factors. A thorough exploration of the etiology and triggers is essential for a comprehensive understanding of epilepsy and for devising targeted strategies for seizure management.

Etiology

A. Genetic Factors

Certain forms of epilepsy have a genetic component, with specific genetic mutations predisposing individuals to seizure disorders. A comprehensive family history assessment and genetic testing can offer insights into the hereditary aspects of epilepsy, facilitating early diagnosis and genetic counseling.

Hereditary Predisposition: Genetic factors contribute substantially to the risk of developing epilepsy. Individuals with a family history of epilepsy are often at an elevated risk, highlighting the hereditary nature of certain forms of the disorder. Recognizing familial patterns is essential for early identification and intervention.

Specific Gene Mutations: Certain gene mutations have been identified as key contributors to epilepsy. These mutations can alter the normal functioning of ion channels, neurotransmitter receptors, or other critical components involved in neuronal excitability. As a result, individuals with specific genetic mutations may have an increased susceptibility to seizures.

Complex Inheritance Patterns: Epilepsy exhibits a diverse range of inheritance patterns, including autosomal dominant, autosomal recessive, and X-linked patterns. Understanding these inheritance mechanisms aids in predicting the likelihood of epilepsy in family members and guides genetic counseling for individuals and their relatives.

Syndromic and Non-Syndromic Epilepsies: Genetic factors contribute to both syndromic and non-syndromic forms of epilepsy. Syndromic epilepsies are characterized by additional features, such as intellectual disabilities or physical abnormalities, alongside seizures. Non-syndromic epilepsies involve seizures as the primary manifestation without associated features. Genetic testing can help distinguish between these categories.

Pharmacogenetics in Antiepileptic Drug Response: Genetic variations also play a role in an individual's response to antiepileptic medications. Pharmacogenetic considerations involve assessing how a person's genetic makeup influences the efficacy and side effects of specific medications. Tailoring treatment plans based on genetic profiles can enhance therapeutic outcomes.

Polygenic Risk: In many cases, epilepsy is polygenic, meaning that multiple genes collectively contribute to an individual's overall risk.

The interplay of various genetic factors, each exerting a modest influence, contributes to the complexity of epilepsy's genetic landscape. Studying polygenic risk enhances our understanding of the disorder's heterogeneity.

Genetic Testing and Counseling: Advances in genetic testing technologies have enabled the identification of specific gene mutations associated with epilepsy. Genetic testing plays a crucial role in confirming diagnoses, guiding treatment decisions, and offering prognostic information. Genetic counseling is essential to help individuals and families understand the implications of genetic findings and make informed decisions about their healthcare.

Understanding the genetic factors as etiological contributors to epilepsy is a dynamic field that continues to evolve with ongoing research. Genetic insights not only enhance our understanding of the disorder's origins but also pave the way for personalized medicine, allowing for tailored interventions that consider an individual's unique genetic makeup. As genetic research progresses, it holds the promise of unlocking new therapeutic avenues and refining our ability to predict, prevent, and manage epilepsy.

B. Structural Brain Abnormalities

Epilepsy often finds its roots in a complex interplay of factors, and structural brain abnormalities stand out as prominent contributors to the disorder's etiology. Understanding how irregularities in the brain's structure can lead to epileptic seizures is essential for accurate diagnosis, targeted interventions, and the provision of comprehensive care.

Tumors and Neoplastic Growth: Tumors within the brain can disrupt normal neuronal activity, leading to the development of epilepsy. These growths may exert pressure on surrounding brain tissue or directly interfere with neural circuits. Recognizing the presence of tumors through advanced imaging techniques like MRI is pivotal for understanding the structural basis of epilepsy.

Developmental Malformations: Anomalies in brain development, occurring either in utero or during early childhood, can contribute to epilepsy. Conditions such as cortical dysplasia, wherein the normal organization of the brain's outer layer is disrupted, can create a substrate for abnormal electrical activity, leading to seizures.

Post-Traumatic Scarring: Brain injuries resulting from trauma, such as head injuries or concussions, can lead to the formation of scar tissue. This scarring, or gliosis, may disrupt the normal connectivity of neurons and contribute to the development of epilepsy. Understanding the history of traumatic events is crucial in assessing the structural underpinnings of seizures.

Vascular Abnormalities: Abnormalities in blood vessels within the brain, such as arteriovenous malformations (AVMs) or aneurysms, can disrupt the flow of blood and oxygen, impacting neuronal function. Structural defects in the vascular system can create conditions conducive to seizures and must be considered in the diagnostic evaluation.

Infections and Inflammatory Processes: Infections affecting the central nervous system, such as encephalitis or meningitis, can lead to inflammation and structural changes. These alterations in brain tissue may create an environment conducive to epileptic activity. Timely identification and treatment of infectious etiologies are essential in managing epilepsy arising from such structural abnormalities.

Genetic Syndromes with Structural Implications: Certain genetic syndromes are associated with structural brain abnormalities that predispose individuals to epilepsy. For example, individuals with tuberous sclerosis complex may develop benign tumors in various organs, including the brain, leading to an increased risk of seizures.

Hippocampal Sclerosis: Hippocampal sclerosis, characterized by damage or atrophy of the hippocampus, is a common structural abnormality observed in individuals with epilepsy, particularly in temporal lobe epilepsy. This structural change disrupts the normal functioning of the hippocampus, a crucial region for memory and spatial navigation, contributing to seizure development.

Advanced neuroimaging technologies, coupled with a thorough clinical history, enable healthcare professionals to identify and characterize these structural anomalies, guiding treatment decisions and enhancing our understanding of epilepsy's diverse origins. As research continues to unravel the intricate relationship between brain structure and epileptogenesis, it holds the promise of advancing our ability to precisely diagnose, treat, and potentially prevent epilepsy stemming from structural abnormalities.

C. Neurochemical Imbalances

Disturbances in neurotransmitter levels, particularly involving gamma-aminobutyric acid (GABA) and glutamate, are implicated in epilepsy. Delving into the intricacies of neurotransmitter dynamics, ion channel function, and genetic contributions reveals the multifaceted nature of neurochemical imbalances in the genesis of epileptic seizures.

GABA and Glutamate Dysregulation: The balance between inhibitory GABAergic and excitatory glutamatergic signaling is crucial for maintaining neuronal equilibrium. Dysregulation in this delicate balance can stem from alterations in receptor density, impaired synthesis or degradation, and disruptions in the reuptake of these neurotransmitters. Consequently, an aberrant GABA/glutamate balance may lower the seizure threshold and contribute to epileptogenesis.

Ion Channel Abnormalities: Ion channels, acting as gatekeepers for neuronal excitability, are integral to neurotransmission. Abnormalities in ion channels, such as sodium, potassium, or calcium channels, can result in disrupted action potentials and contribute to hyperexcitability. Genetic mutations or acquired channelopathies may lead to persistent depolarization, making neurons more prone to firing spontaneously.

Altered Neurotransmitter Receptor Function: Neurotransmitters exert their effects by binding to specific receptors, initiating downstream signaling cascades. Changes in receptor density, affinity, or post-translational modifications can impact receptor function. For instance, alterations in GABA receptor function, whether due to genetic factors or acquired changes, may compromise inhibitory control, facilitating seizure generation.

Neurotransmitter Metabolism: The intricate orchestration of neurotransmitter synthesis, release, and degradation contributes to their precise regulation. Enzymatic deficiencies or disruptions in these processes can lead to imbalances, impacting the availability of neurotransmitters critical for maintaining neuronal stability.

Neurotransmitter Transporter Aberrations: Transporters play a vital role in the reuptake and recycling of neurotransmitters. Dysregulation in these processes can prolong the presence of neurotransmitters in the synaptic cleft, leading to sustained signaling and potential hyperexcitability. Genetic variations or acquired changes in transporter function may contribute to this dysregulation.

Neurotransmitter Modulation by Hormones: Hormones influence neurotransmitter dynamics, adding another layer of complexity to epileptogenesis. Fluctuations in hormonal levels during different phases of the menstrual cycle, pregnancy, or menopause can modulate neurotransmitter release and receptor sensitivity, influencing the threshold for seizure activity.

Genetic Contributions to Neurotransmitter Dynamics: Genetic factors influence various facets of neurotransmission, from receptor structure to enzyme function. Polymorphisms or mutations in genes coding for key players in neurotransmitter dynamics can predispose individuals to epilepsy. Understanding the genetic landscape provides insights into personalized treatment approaches targeting specific neurochemical aberrations.

This intricate understanding of neurochemical imbalances not only informs the development of antiepileptic medications but also lays the foundation for precision medicine in epilepsy. Targeting specific neurotransmitter systems, ion channels, or genetic factors associated with neurochemical dysregulation holds promise for more effective and tailored therapeutic interventions.

As research in neurochemistry advances, it opens avenues for unraveling the nuances of neurochemical imbalances in epilepsy, ultimately leading to a more comprehensive understanding of the disorder and fostering the development of innovative treatments that address its diverse etiological underpinnings.

D. Developmental Disorders

Certain developmental disorders, including autism spectrum disorders, have associations with an increased risk of epilepsy. Recognizing these associations early in life enables a more comprehensive approach to care, addressing both developmental and epileptic aspects.

Autism Spectrum Disorders (ASD): Individuals with ASD often face an increased risk of epilepsy. The association between ASD and epilepsy is complex, involving shared genetic factors and abnormalities in brain development. Early recognition of ASD symptoms, coupled with vigilant monitoring for seizure activity, is crucial for timely intervention and tailored management.

Intellectual Disabilities: Intellectual disabilities, often co-occurring with epilepsy, underscore the intricate interplay between cognitive function and seizure susceptibility. Developmental challenges affecting intellectual abilities may result from genetic syndromes, structural brain abnormalities, or other factors, contributing to the overall complexity of epilepsy etiology.

Cerebral Palsy: Cerebral palsy, a group of disorders affecting movement and posture, is frequently associated with epilepsy. Brain injuries during prenatal or perinatal development, leading to cerebral palsy, may create a neurodevelopmental milieu conducive to epileptic seizures. Multidisciplinary care is essential to address the complex needs of individuals with both conditions.

Genetic Syndromes with Developmental Implications: Several genetic syndromes characterized by developmental abnormalities are linked to an increased risk of epilepsy. Examples include Down syndrome, Rett syndrome, and Angelman syndrome. The genetic underpinnings of these syndromes contribute to both developmental challenges and an elevated susceptibility to seizures.

Fetal Alcohol Spectrum Disorders (FASD): Exposure to alcohol during prenatal development can lead to a spectrum of disorders known as FASD, encompassing a range of physical, cognitive, and behavioral impairments. Individuals with FASD may experience an increased likelihood of epilepsy, emphasizing the importance of preventive measures and early intervention.

Neonatal Seizures and Brain Injury: Seizures occurring in the neonatal period, often associated with brain injury, can have long-term implications for development and increase the risk of epilepsy. Identifying and addressing the underlying causes of neonatal seizures, such as hypoxic-ischemic events or infections, is crucial for mitigating the risk of subsequent epilepsy.

Environmental Exposures and Neurodevelopment: Certain environmental exposures during critical periods of neurodevelopment may contribute to both developmental disorders and epilepsy. Factors such as prenatal exposure to toxins, infections, or trauma can influence the trajectory of brain development, creating conditions conducive to the later onset of epilepsy.

Understanding developmental disorders as etiological foundations of epilepsy requires a holistic approach that considers the intertwined nature of neurological and cognitive development. Early identification of developmental challenges, coupled with vigilant monitoring for seizure activity, allows for tailored interventions that address the unique needs of individuals navigating the complex intersection of developmental disorders and epilepsy.

E. Infections and Inflammatory Conditions

Epilepsy often draws its origins from a myriad of factors, with infections and inflammatory conditions standing out as influential contributors. The dynamic interplay between the immune system and the central nervous system is complex, and understanding how infections and inflammation contribute to epileptogenesis is crucial for nuanced diagnostics, targeted interventions, and holistic patient care.

Encephalitis: Encephalitis, whether caused by viral infections or triggered by autoimmune responses, is a recognized precursor to epilepsy. The inflammatory processes within the brain during encephalitis can result in acute seizures and lay the groundwork for long-term epileptic tendencies. Distinguishing between infectious and autoimmune encephalitis is essential for tailoring treatment strategies and anticipating the potential for recurrent seizures.

Meningitis: Meningitis, characterized by inflammation of the membranes surrounding the brain and spinal cord, poses a significant risk for seizures. Both bacterial and viral forms of meningitis can lead to neurological complications, including epilepsy. Swift diagnosis and targeted treatment are imperative to mitigate the neurological consequences and reduce the likelihood of epilepsy development.

HIV-Associated Neurological Complications: Individuals living with human immunodeficiency virus (HIV) are susceptible to neurological complications, with seizures being a potential manifestation. HIV-associated encephalitis or opportunistic infections affecting the central nervous system can contribute to the development of epilepsy. Managing epilepsy in the context of HIV requires a comprehensive approach addressing both virological control and neurological manifestations.

Infections in Neonates: Neonatal infections, particularly those that involve the central nervous system, can have profound implications for neurological development and increase the risk of epilepsy. Timely recognition and intervention to treat infections in neonates are pivotal in preventing long-term neurological sequelae, including the development of epilepsy.

Inflammatory Disorders: Chronic inflammatory conditions, such as systemic lupus erythematosus or rheumatoid arthritis, may extend their impact on the central nervous system, leading to seizures. Inflammatory processes affecting the brain parenchyma or blood vessels can contribute to the development of epilepsy in individuals with these autoimmune disorders. Managing epilepsy in the context of chronic inflammatory conditions requires a comprehensive understanding of the underlying disease mechanisms.

Post-Infectious Epilepsy: Seizures may persist as a consequence of previous infections, even after the infection has been successfully treated. The lingering impact of the immune response and inflammatory changes during the infection may create an environment conducive to the development of epilepsy. Post-infectious epilepsy highlights the importance of long-term monitoring and management strategies beyond the resolution of the initial infection.

Diagnostic evaluation involves not only identifying the specific infectious agent or autoimmune process but also understanding the extent of immune-mediated damage and its implications for neurological function. Treatment strategies encompass antiviral medications, immunomodulatory therapies, and anti-inflammatory agents based on the underlying cause.

Multidisciplinary collaboration among neurologists, infectious disease specialists, and immunologists is essential for managing epilepsy arising from infections and inflammatory conditions. Beyond acute interventions, long-term strategies focus on preventing recurrent seizures, mitigating the impact of immune responses on the brain, and optimizing the overall quality of life for individuals navigating the complex intersection of infections, inflammation, and epilepsy.

Triggers

Sleep Deprivation: Lack of sufficient or irregular sleep patterns has a profound impact on seizure susceptibility by lowering the seizure threshold. The intricate relationship between sleep and epilepsy underscores the importance of incorporating healthy sleep hygiene practices. Establishing consistent sleep routines, maintaining a conducive sleep environment, and addressing sleep disorders are integral components of seizure management. Moreover, recognizing individual variations in the relationship between sleep and seizures allows for personalized strategies to optimize sleep-related seizure control.

Stress and Emotional Factors: Emotional stress, anxiety, and psychological factors can act as potent triggers for seizures, emphasizing the intricate connection between the mind and seizures. Implementing stress management techniques is crucial in mitigating seizure risk. Psychotherapeutic interventions, mindfulness practices, relaxation exercises, and cognitive-behavioral therapy contribute to psychological well-being and play a pivotal role in seizure control. Tailoring stress management strategies to individual preferences and needs empowers individuals to navigate emotional challenges effectively, reducing the impact on seizure frequency.

Sensory Stimuli: Certain sensory stimuli, such as flashing lights (photosensitivity), specific patterns, or loud noises, can provoke seizures in susceptible individuals. Identifying and avoiding these triggers whenever possible is essential. Adaptive strategies, including wearing tinted glasses or using filters on electronic devices, can help mitigate the impact of sensory stimuli on seizure occurrence. Understanding the individual's unique sensitivities to sensory triggers allows for personalized interventions that enhance overall seizure management.

Medication Non-Adherence: Inconsistent or incorrect use of antiepileptic medications poses a significant risk for breakthrough seizures. Patient education on the importance of medication adherence is paramount. Regular medication reviews, collaborative discussions with healthcare providers, and open communication about potential side effects contribute to optimizing seizure control. Tailored medication regimens, considering individual preferences and lifestyle factors, enhance adherence and minimize the risk of medication-related breakthrough seizures.

Hormonal Changes: Hormonal fluctuations, particularly in women during menstruation, pregnancy, or menopause, exert a notable influence on seizure frequency. Tailoring treatment plans to account for hormonal changes involves adjusting medication dosages and implementing hormonal management strategies. A collaborative approach between individuals, healthcare providers, and specialists in reproductive health ensures comprehensive care that addresses the dynamic interplay between hormones and seizures.

Alcohol and Substance Abuse: Excessive alcohol consumption or substance abuse significantly lowers the seizure threshold, making individuals more susceptible to seizures. Integrating substance abuse counseling, participation in support groups, and access to rehabilitation services are essential components of epilepsy care. These interventions not only address modifiable risk factors but also contribute to overall health and well-being.

Specific Triggers for Certain Epilepsy Syndromes: Recognizing specific triggers associated with certain epilepsy syndromes allows for targeted anticipatory guidance and preventive measures. For example, individuals with febrile seizure syndromes may be prone to seizures during febrile illnesses. Understanding syndrome-specific triggers enables healthcare providers to tailor interventions, including fever management strategies and timely adjustments to treatment plans, to enhance overall seizure control.

Understanding the multifaceted etiology of epilepsy, including genetic predisposition, structural considerations, and neurochemical dynamics, provides a foundation for comprehensive care. Equally important is the recognition and management of individual triggers, empowering individuals with epilepsy to actively engage in their care and optimize their overall quality of life.

Social and Cultural Perceptions

Epilepsy exists at the intersection of medical challenges and societal perceptions. The social and cultural landscape plays a crucial role in shaping the experiences of individuals with epilepsy, influencing how the condition is viewed and understood within communities. A detailed exploration of social and cultural perceptions unveils a nuanced tapestry of historical contexts, prevailing attitudes, and persistent misconceptions.

Historical Perspectives: Tracing the historical roots of societal perceptions reveals diverse cultural interpretations of epilepsy. Ancient societies often associated seizures with mystical or supernatural forces, perpetuating stigma and marginalization. Analyzing these historical lenses provides valuable insights into the origins of societal attitudes and guides efforts to reshape perceptions in contemporary contexts.

Stigma and Discrimination: Epilepsy stigma persists as a formidable barrier, leading to discrimination, social exclusion, and profound challenges. Prevailing misconceptions about the contagious nature of epilepsy or unfounded fears regarding violence during seizures contribute to societal stigmatization. Robust educational campaigns that debunk myths and emphasize the normalcy of daily life for individuals with epilepsy are essential for dismantling pervasive stigma.

Cultural Beliefs and Traditions: Cultural beliefs and traditions exert a significant influence on how epilepsy is perceived. Certain cultures attribute seizures to supernatural forces, karma, or divine punishment. Recognizing and respecting these cultural nuances is crucial for developing culturally sensitive approaches to epilepsy education, awareness, and advocacy.

Impact on Education and Employment: Societal perceptions translate into tangible consequences, affecting education and

35

employment opportunities for individuals with epilepsy. Misconceptions about cognitive abilities and workplace safety can lead to discrimination. Advocacy for inclusive educational environments and workplace accommodations is vital for breaking down systemic barriers and promoting equal opportunities.

Advocacy and Awareness Campaigns: Addressing societal attitudes requires sustained advocacy and awareness campaigns. These initiatives aim to dispel myths, challenge stereotypes, and disseminate accurate information about epilepsy. Collaborative efforts involving healthcare professionals, advocacy organizations, and individuals with epilepsy contribute to reshaping societal narratives and fostering understanding.

Healthcare Disparities: Social and cultural perceptions influence healthcare disparities experienced by individuals with epilepsy. Stigmatization may result in delays in seeking medical help, and cultural taboos may affect the acceptance of medical interventions. Culturally competent healthcare practices, coupled with targeted outreach programs, are essential for overcoming these barriers and ensuring equitable healthcare access.

Empowering the Epilepsy Community: Empowering individuals with epilepsy involves creating platforms for them to share their stories and advocate for change. Personal narratives humanize the condition, challenge stereotypes, and inspire empathy. The establishment of peer support networks and community engagement initiatives plays a vital role in fostering a sense of belonging and challenging societal misconceptions.

Legislation and Policy Advocacy: Legal frameworks and policies play a pivotal role in addressing discrimination and safeguarding the rights of individuals with epilepsy. Advocacy efforts focus on ensuring equal access to education, employment, healthcare, and public spaces. Collaborative initiatives between advocacy groups and policymakers contribute to the development of inclusive policies that protect the rights and dignity of those with epilepsy.

Global Perspectives and Cultural Competence: Acknowledging the global diversity of perceptions surrounding epilepsy is imperative. Cultural competence in epilepsy care involves tailoring educational materials, interventions, and support systems to align with cultural contexts. Cross-cultural understanding fosters respectful and inclusive approaches that bridge gaps in knowledge and foster acceptance on a global scale.

In conclusion, unraveling the intricate fabric of social and cultural perceptions surrounding epilepsy demands a comprehensive and multi-faceted approach. Education, advocacy, and policy changes are pivotal in challenging misconceptions, dismantling stigma, and fostering environments where individuals with epilepsy can thrive. Embracing diversity, promoting empathy, and amplifying the voices of those affected by epilepsy contribute to the creation of a more inclusive and understanding society.

Chapter Two: Diagnosis and Treatment Options

This chapter explores diagnostic intricacies and diverse treatment modalities. Beginning with a detailed examination of diagnostic procedures, it unravels crucial steps for accurate epilepsy diagnosis. Navigating through medical treatments, diverse interventions, and their efficacy in seizure control are discussed. The exploration extends to surgical options, illuminating various treatments and their outcomes. Beyond conventional approaches, holistic perspectives are embraced, exploring complementary and alternative methods for epilepsy management. This chapter aims to provide nuanced insights into diagnostics and treatments, equipping readers with a comprehensive understanding of epilepsy's landscape.

Diagnostic Procedures

Achieving an accurate diagnosis of epilepsy entails a meticulous process designed to unravel the complexities of seizure disorders, identify their root causes, and pave the way for effective treatment strategies. This comprehensive journey involves several detailed steps:

Clinical History and Seizure Description

Clinical history and seizure description form the initial pillars of the diagnostic process for epilepsy, providing clinicians with essential insights into the nature and context of seizures. During the clinical history assessment, healthcare professionals delve into the individual's medical background, seeking information about any previous episodes suggestive of seizures.

This involves a detailed inquiry into the onset, duration, and frequency of seizures, as well as associated symptoms or triggers. The seizure description is a critical component, requiring individuals to articulate their experiences during seizure events. Details such as the type of movements, alterations in consciousness, and any preictal or postictal phenomena are meticulously recorded.

Additionally, factors like potential triggers, environmental circumstances, and the presence of aura are explored. This collaborative process between healthcare providers and individuals ensures a comprehensive understanding of the seizure manifestations, guiding subsequent diagnostic investigations and personalized treatment strategies.

Physical Examination

The physical examination is a fundamental aspect of diagnosing epilepsy, extending beyond routine assessments to focus on neurological signs and abnormalities. During this examination, healthcare professionals carefully evaluate various aspects of the individual's physical health, with a specific emphasis on neurological function.

Neurological examinations include assessing motor function, reflexes, sensory responses, and coordination. Clinicians may observe for any abnormal movements, muscle tone irregularities, or signs of neurological dysfunction. This thorough evaluation aims to identify subtle indicators that might be associated with epilepsy or neurological conditions.

By combining clinical history, seizure description, and a comprehensive physical examination, healthcare providers can gather valuable information to guide further diagnostic investigations and ensure a holistic understanding of the individual's condition.

Electroencephalogram (EEG)

The Electroencephalogram (EEG) is a pivotal diagnostic tool used in the assessment of epilepsy. It records and measures the electrical activity generated by the brain, providing valuable insights into its functioning. This non-invasive procedure involves attaching electrodes to the scalp, which detect and amplify the electrical signals produced by neurons.

EEG readings help identify abnormal patterns indicative of epilepsy, such as spikes, sharp waves, or other irregularities. The test is particularly valuable for capturing the brain's activity during and between seizures. Prolonged EEG monitoring, sometimes performed over several days, enhances the chances of capturing elusive seizure events, contributing to a more accurate diagnosis and informing tailored treatment plans. EEGs play a crucial role in confirming the presence of epilepsy and determining its specific characteristics.

Imaging Studies (MRI and CT scans)

Imaging studies, specifically Magnetic Resonance Imaging (MRI) and Computed Tomography (CT) scans, play a pivotal role in the diagnostic process for epilepsy. These non-invasive techniques provide detailed images of the brain's structure, aiding clinicians in identifying any abnormalities or lesions that may contribute to seizures.

Magnetic Resonance Imaging (MRI): MRI utilizes powerful magnets and radio waves to generate detailed images of the brain's soft tissues. It is particularly effective in visualizing structural abnormalities, such as tumors, vascular malformations, or scarring, which might be associated with epilepsy. The high-resolution and multi-dimensional views offered by MRI contribute to precise diagnostic insights.

Computed Tomography (CT) Scan: CT scans involve X-rays to create cross-sectional images of the brain. While they are valuable for detecting gross abnormalities, CT scans may be less detailed than MRIs in visualizing soft tissues. CT scans are often used in emergencies or when MRI is contraindicated.

These imaging studies are essential components of the diagnostic journey, providing clinicians with a comprehensive view of the brain's anatomy. The information gleaned from MRI and CT scans assists in confirming epilepsy diagnoses, identifying structural causes, and guiding appropriate treatment strategies tailored to the individual's specific condition.

Blood Tests

Blood tests are integral in the diagnostic process for epilepsy, aiding in the identification of various factors that could be linked to seizures. These tests involve analyzing blood samples to assess different parameters relevant to epilepsy diagnosis and management.

Metabolic Tests: Metabolic blood tests help identify imbalances in electrolytes, glucose levels, or other metabolic markers that might trigger seizures or indicate underlying metabolic disorders.

Genetic Testing: Genetic blood tests, particularly in cases with a family history of epilepsy, focus on identifying specific genetic mutations or variations associated with seizure disorders. These tests offer insights into the genetic underpinnings of epilepsy and guide treatment decisions.

Drug Levels: Monitoring antiepileptic drug levels in the blood is essential to ensure therapeutic concentrations. Blood tests help determine if the prescribed medications are within the effective range and aid in adjusting dosages if needed.

Infectious Diseases and Autoimmune Markers: Blood tests may also screen for infectious diseases or autoimmune markers that could contribute to seizures. Identifying these underlying conditions assists in formulating appropriate treatment plans.

These blood tests complement other diagnostic procedures, offering valuable information to clinicians in confirming an epilepsy diagnosis, ruling out underlying conditions, and guiding personalized treatment approaches tailored to the individual's specific needs.

Video EEG Monitoring:

Video EEG Monitoring represents an advanced diagnostic method in epilepsy assessment, combining conventional EEG recording with simultaneous video surveillance. This holistic approach provides clinicians with synchronized insights into both brain activity and the individual's behavior during seizure events. The continuous video component allows for a comprehensive observation of an individual's movements, gestures, and visible signs alongside the corresponding EEG patterns.

This amalgamation of visual and electrical data enhances diagnostic accuracy, enabling a more nuanced understanding of different seizure types, and aiding in classification and characterization. Beyond mere observation, Video EEG Monitoring offers a prolonged monitoring period, facilitating the assessment of seizure frequency, duration, and potential triggers.

This extended observation is crucial in identifying triggers and patterns that may contribute to seizures. Furthermore, the comprehensive recording includes sleep and wake cycles, shedding light on how these states influence seizure occurrence. This detailed information contributes significantly to tailoring treatment plans and understanding the impact of different physiological states on seizure activity.

Neuropsychological Testing

Neuropsychological testing is an essential facet of the epilepsy diagnostic process, offering profound insights into the cognitive and psychological dimensions of an individual's condition. This specialized evaluation systematically assesses various cognitive functions, providing a detailed profile that includes memory, processing speed, and problem-solving abilities. Moreover, it delves

45

into how seizures may impact daily functioning, shedding light on the intricate interplay between epilepsy and cognitive performance.

Beyond simply identifying cognitive impairments associated with epilepsy, these assessments differentiate them from the direct effects of seizures and medications, allowing for more targeted treatment planning. The results gleaned from neuropsychological testing play a pivotal role in tailoring holistic treatment plans. This may involve cognitive rehabilitation, counseling, or educational support, addressing specific cognitive challenges and contributing to overall well-being.

Furthermore, neuropsychological assessments offer valuable prognostic information, enabling clinicians to anticipate potential challenges and tailor long-term management strategies for individuals navigating life with epilepsy. By providing a comprehensive understanding of the cognitive impact of seizures, neuropsychological testing becomes a cornerstone in the diagnostic journey, guiding nuanced interventions and fostering holistic approaches to epilepsy.

Genetic Testing

The primary objective of genetic testing is to pinpoint specific mutations or variations in genes associated with epilepsy. This not only confirms a genetic basis for the condition but also sheds light on the potential hereditary aspects, informing both clinicians and individuals about the origin of their seizures. Understanding the genetic underpinnings allows for a more nuanced approach to prognosis, enabling healthcare professionals to anticipate the trajectory of the condition and tailor management strategies accordingly.

Moreover, genetic testing contributes significantly to personalized treatment approaches. By revealing the specific genetic factors at play, healthcare providers can tailor interventions that align with the underlying genetic mechanisms. This targeted approach enhances the efficacy of treatment strategies, optimizing the chances of successful seizure management.

The implications of genetic testing extend beyond the individual, influencing family planning and counseling. Positive findings may prompt genetic counseling, empowering individuals and their families to make informed decisions about family planning and better comprehend the potential hereditary risk of epilepsy within the family.

Specialized Testing (PET and SPECT scans)

Specialized imaging studies, namely Positron Emission Tomography (PET) and Single Photon Emission Computed Tomography (SPECT) scans, play a pivotal role in the intricate diagnostic evaluation of epilepsy.

Positron Emission Tomography (PET) scans offer unique insights into brain activity by detecting regions with altered metabolic rates. Through the injection of a trace amount of radioactive material, PET scans illuminate areas of heightened or diminished metabolic activity, aiding in the precise localization of abnormal brain function associated with epilepsy. This functional perspective proves invaluable, especially when structural abnormalities may not be immediately evident.

Single Photon Emission Computed Tomography (SPECT) scans provide complementary functional information by capturing the distribution of a radiotracer injected into the bloodstream. They excel in identifying areas of abnormal blood flow or metabolic activity associated with seizure foci. SPECT scans serve as a crucial tool when seeking to understand functional disturbances that may underlie seizures, even in the absence of clear structural anomalies.

Both play a vital role in cases where traditional imaging falls short, providing essential data to locate seizure foci, guide treatment decisions, and, in some cases, determine the suitability of surgical interventions. These advanced imaging studies enhance diagnostics, offering a more comprehensive understanding of epilepsy's neurobiological intricacies and aiding in the development of personalized therapeutic strategies for individuals living with epilepsy.

Seizure Diary and Patient Input

Maintaining a seizure diary and incorporating patient input are essential components of epilepsy management. A seizure diary involves the systematic recording of details related to seizures, including their frequency, duration, and any associated factors or triggers. This tool not only assists healthcare professionals in tracking the course of the condition but also empowers individuals to actively participate in their care.

Patient input, comprising firsthand accounts of seizure experiences, is invaluable in providing qualitative insights that may not be captured through medical tests alone. Descriptions of seizure auras, postictal states, and the impact on daily life contribute to a holistic understanding of the individual's experience with epilepsy.

The combination of a seizure diary and patient input enhances the diagnostic process, aids in treatment decision-making, and enables personalized care. It fosters a collaborative relationship between healthcare providers and individuals with epilepsy, ensuring a more comprehensive and tailored approach to managing the condition.

By methodically navigating through these diagnostic procedures, clinicians can unravel the intricate tapestry of epilepsy. This meticulous approach not only ensures an accurate diagnosis but also lays the foundation for tailored treatment plans, empowering individuals with epilepsy to manage their condition effectively.

Medical Treatments

Epilepsy management necessitates a comprehensive understanding of various medical interventions, each tailored to the unique aspects of an individual's condition. A thorough examination of these treatments offers valuable insights into how they work and their efficacy, playing a role in enhancing the management of seizures. In the following sections, we take a closer look at essential medical interventions:

Antiepileptic Medications (AEDs)

Antiepileptic medications (AEDs) stand as the foremost pharmacological intervention in the intricate landscape of epilepsy management. Their fundamental role lies in modulating neuronal activity and mitigating abnormal electrical discharges that precipitate seizures. The array of available AEDs offers healthcare providers a nuanced toolkit to tailor treatment strategies to the individual characteristics of each patient.

One of the key aspects of understanding AEDs is their diverse mechanisms of action. These medications exert their influence by targeting neurotransmitters or ion channels, stabilizing neuronal membranes, and averting the hyperexcitability that underlies seizures. The specificity of these mechanisms allows for targeted interventions based on the unique neurobiological factors at play in each patient.

AEDs can be broadly categorized into two types: broad-spectrum and narrow-spectrum. The former, exemplified by valproic acid and lamotrigine, addresses a wide range of seizure types. In contrast, narrow-spectrum AEDs like ethosuximide are more selective, proving effective against specific seizure types.

The choice between monotherapy and polytherapy, involving a single drug or a combination, is contingent upon the patient's response and seizure persistence. This decision-making process considers factors such as compatibility between medications and their synergistic effects.

Initiating and titrating AEDs involves a meticulous assessment of patient variables, including age, overall health, and seizure type. This iterative process aims to achieve optimal seizure control while minimizing potential side effects. Close monitoring during initiation and titration is essential to determine the most effective and well-tolerated dosage.

While AEDs are paramount in seizure management, they are not without side effects. Ranging from mild to severe, common side effects include drowsiness, dizziness, and gastrointestinal disturbances. A collaborative approach between healthcare providers and patients addresses these side effects, with adjustments made to medication regimens if necessary. Regular monitoring, including blood tests to measure medication levels, ensures that therapeutic ranges are maintained for optimal seizure control.

The journey with AEDs is inherently individualized, necessitating tailored treatment plans. Factors such as age, comorbidities, and lifestyle considerations shape the selection of medications. Regular reevaluation allows healthcare providers to make adjustments based on the evolving needs of the patient.

Beyond their physical impact, AEDs have psychosocial implications. Cognitive effects, mood changes, and concerns about medication adherence are acknowledged and managed collaboratively to ensure holistic care.

Medical Marijuana (Cannabidiol)

Medical marijuana, specifically Cannabidiol (CBD), has emerged as a noteworthy subject of exploration in the realm of epilepsy management. CBD, a non-psychoactive compound derived from the cannabis plant, has garnered attention for its potential as an adjunct therapy for certain epilepsy syndromes, particularly those resistant to conventional treatments.

The mechanism through which CBD exerts its antiseizure effects is not entirely understood but is thought to involve interactions with the endocannabinoid system, impacting neurotransmitter signaling and neuronal excitability. CBD differs from tetrahydrocannabinol (THC), another cannabis-derived compound known for its psychoactive effects, as it does not induce euphoria or intoxication.

FDA-approved CBD medications, such as Epidiolex, have been developed for specific epilepsy syndromes, notably Dravet syndrome and Lennox-Gastaut syndrome. Clinical trials have demonstrated promising results, showing a reduction in seizure frequency among patients receiving CBD treatment.

While CBD holds promise as an antiseizure agent, it is important to note that its use requires careful consideration and medical supervision. The dosage, purity, and consistency of CBD products can vary, emphasizing the need for standardized formulations and rigorous quality control measures. Additionally, potential interactions with other medications must be carefully evaluated.

CBD's therapeutic scope extends beyond seizure control, showing potential in managing comorbidities associated with epilepsy, such as sleep disturbances and behavioral issues. Ongoing research endeavors seek to explore its broader applications, elucidate its long-term effects, and identify optimal dosing regimens.

As with any medical intervention, the decision to incorporate CBD into an epilepsy treatment plan involves discussions between healthcare providers and patients. Open dialogue, comprehensive assessments, and diligent monitoring are crucial aspects of integrating CBD as part of a holistic approach to epilepsy management, ensuring patient safety and optimizing therapeutic outcomes.

In essence, the exploration of Cannabidiol as a potential therapeutic agent signifies a novel avenue in epilepsy care. Its distinct properties and promising antiseizure effects highlight the ongoing evolution and diversification of treatment modalities, offering individuals with epilepsy and their healthcare teams an additional tool in their pursuit of optimal seizure control and improved quality of life.

Adapting Medications for Women

Recognizing the intricate interplay between hormonal fluctuations and epilepsy, the adaptation of medications for women emerges as a crucial consideration in providing personalized and effective care. Women's hormonal cycles, influenced by menstruation, pregnancy, and menopause, can significantly impact seizure frequency and intensity. Tailoring medication strategies to account for these fluctuations is essential for optimizing seizure control.

Seizure patterns often exhibit variability across the menstrual cycle, with hormonal changes during the premenstrual phase potentially influencing seizure susceptibility. Healthcare providers work collaboratively with women to identify patterns and adjust medication dosages as needed during specific phases of the menstrual cycle.

For women of childbearing age, considerations extend to pregnancy planning and management. Certain antiepileptic medications may pose risks during pregnancy, impacting fetal development. Healthcare providers engage in proactive discussions about family planning, and adjusting medications as needed to minimize risks while maintaining optimal seizure control.

Pregnancy introduces dynamic hormonal shifts that can influence the pharmacokinetics of antiepileptic medications. Regular monitoring and adjustments are made to ensure that medication levels remain within therapeutic ranges. This adaptive approach is crucial for balancing the well-being of both the expectant mother and the developing fetus.

The postpartum period brings its own set of hormonal changes. Medication adjustments made during pregnancy may need further modification after childbirth. Close monitoring and open communication with healthcare providers ensure that any necessary adaptations are made to support the woman's evolving needs.

Menopause represents another phase where hormonal fluctuations may impact seizure control. Adjustments to antiepileptic medications are considered to address the potential influence of hormonal changes during this life stage.

Every woman's experience with epilepsy is unique, necessitating individualized treatment plans. Factors such as age, overall health, and lifestyle considerations are integral components in crafting medication strategies that effectively navigate hormonal influences while optimizing overall well-being.

The adaptability of medication strategies for women with epilepsy underscores the importance of a collaborative and patient-centered approach. Regular communication, comprehensive assessments, and a willingness to adjust treatment plans based on individual responses contribute to a more personalized and effective management of epilepsy in women across different life stages. In essence, the nuanced consideration of hormonal influences ensures that medication strategies align with the specific needs and experiences of women living with epilepsy.

Treatments for Specific Epilepsy Syndromes

Epilepsy encompasses a spectrum of syndromes, each presenting with distinctive features and requiring tailored treatment strategies to effectively manage seizures and associated challenges.

Childhood Absence Epilepsy, characterized by brief lapses in consciousness, often responds well to antiepileptic medications like ethosuximide, valproic acid, or lamotrigine. These drugs aim to prevent the specific absence of seizures typical of this syndrome.

Dravet Syndrome, a complex and drug-resistant form of epilepsy, may necessitate a multifaceted approach. Stiripentol, clobazam, and cannabidiol (CBD) have shown promise in reducing seizures, and the ketogenic diet is sometimes explored for its potential benefits.

Lennox-Gastaut Syndrome, marked by multiple seizure types, often requires a combination of antiepileptic medications. Medications such as valproic acid, lamotrigine, and rufinamide may be used. Non-pharmacological interventions, including vagus nerve stimulation (VNS) or responsive neurostimulation (RNS), are additional considerations.

Juvenile Myoclonic Epilepsy (JME) commonly responds to antiepileptic medications like valproic acid. Alternatives such as levetiracetam and lamotrigine may be considered. Long-term management and adherence are crucial components in controlling myoclonic and generalized tonic-clonic seizures associated with JME.

Temporal Lobe Epilepsy, often characterized by complex partial seizures, is typically managed with antiepileptic medications like carbamazepine or lamotrigine. Surgical options, such as temporal lobectomy, may be explored for individuals resistant to medications.

Frontal Lobe Epilepsy may respond to medications such as levetiracetam or oxcarbazepine. However, pinpointing the specific seizure focus is critical for tailored treatment. In cases of drug-resistant frontal lobe epilepsy, surgical interventions, including resective surgery, may be considered.

Benign Rolandic Epilepsy, commonly seen in children, often resolves with age. During the active phase, antiepileptic medications like carbamazepine or oxcarbazepine may be prescribed, with close monitoring for timely adjustments.

Landau-Kleffner Syndrome, affecting language and behavior, may involve corticosteroids and antiepileptic medications like benzodiazepines. Behavioral and speech therapy can complement medical interventions in managing this complex syndrome.

Febrile Seizures, typically occurring in children during fever episodes, often do not require ongoing medication. However, recurrent febrile seizures or the development of Febrile Seizures Plus syndrome may prompt consideration of antiepileptic medications.

Tailoring treatments for specific epilepsy syndromes demands a nuanced understanding of each syndrome's characteristics and the unique aspects of individual patients.

Navigating the realm of medical treatments for epilepsy requires a collaborative effort between healthcare providers and individuals. Regular communication, diligent monitoring, and a willingness to explore different options are paramount. This in-depth understanding of diverse interventions empowers individuals and their healthcare teams to craft personalized treatment plans, optimizing effectiveness while considering the nuanced aspects of epilepsy management.

Surgical Options

Surgical interventions for epilepsy aim to provide long-term seizure control, especially for individuals who do not respond to or tolerate antiepileptic medications. The decision to explore surgical options is typically made after comprehensive evaluations, including imaging studies, electroencephalogram (EEG) monitoring, and neuropsychological assessments. Here, we delve into various surgical options and their outcomes in the management of epilepsy.

Resective Surgery

Resective surgery emerges as a crucial intervention in the realm of epilepsy treatment, particularly for those grappling with focal seizures emanating from identifiable brain regions. This surgical approach involves the targeted removal of specific brain tissue responsible for generating seizures, offering a potential long-term solution when conventional antiepileptic medications prove insufficient.

Before embarking on resective surgery, a comprehensive preoperative evaluation takes place. This involves advanced imaging studies such as magnetic resonance imaging (MRI) to precisely locate the seizure focus. Electroencephalogram (EEG) monitoring complements these studies, providing valuable insights into abnormal brain activity patterns and guiding the surgical planning process. Neurosurgeons collaborate with multidisciplinary teams to determine the optimal surgical approach, which may include procedures like lobectomy, where an entire lobe of the brain is removed, or lesionectomy, targeting specific abnormalities identified in imaging studies. Intraoperative monitoring, including continuous EEG monitoring, ensures real-time assessment of brain activity, enabling the surgical team to delineate between healthy and epileptogenic tissue.

The outcomes of resective surgery are often marked by significant success in reducing seizure frequency or achieving complete seizure freedom, especially for individuals with well-defined seizure foci. Beyond seizure control, successful surgery may contribute to improved cognitive outcomes, particularly in cases where epilepsy originates from regions critical for cognitive function. This is particularly relevant in pediatric cases, where early intervention can positively impact cognitive development and overall quality of life. The benefits extend to an enhanced overall well-being, including improved mood, cognitive clarity, and increased independence.

However, the decision to pursue resective surgery is not without its considerations. Potential risks, such as infection, bleeding, or adverse effects on cognitive function, must be thoroughly discussed between healthcare providers and patients. Additionally, not all individuals with epilepsy are suitable candidates for resective surgery. The decision hinges on factors such as the localization of the seizure focus, the individual's overall health, and the potential impact on cognitive function.

In essence, resective surgery represents a precise and targeted approach to epilepsy management. With advancements in neuroimaging and surgical techniques, this intervention offers renewed hope for individuals whose lives are significantly impacted by seizures. The decision to pursue resective surgery involves careful consideration and collaboration between healthcare providers and patients, ultimately striving for improved seizure control and an enhanced quality of life.

Corpus Callosotomy

Corpus callosotomy serves as a surgical remedy primarily targeted at managing severe and intractable seizures, particularly those originating from a generalized onset that significantly impacts consciousness. This intricate procedure involves the surgical disconnection of the corpus callosum, the vital structure responsible for facilitating communication between the brain's hemispheres.

The process initiates with a comprehensive preoperative assessment that typically encompasses advanced imaging techniques like magnetic resonance imaging (MRI). These imaging studies aid in meticulously visualizing the brain's structural intricacies, precisely identifying potential irregularities or abnormalities contributing to the seizures.

The surgical technique unfolds through a carefully orchestrated series of steps. Surgeons initiate the procedure with a craniotomy, creating an opening in the skull to access the corpus callosum. Subsequently, a strategic severing or partial sectioning of the corpus callosum occurs, disrupting the pathways that facilitate the rapid spread of seizure activity between hemispheres.

Corpus callosotomy often adopts a staged approach, with the surgery performed in incremental disconnections targeting specific regions before ultimately leading to complete sectioning of the corpus callosum. This method allows for a progressive evaluation of the impact on seizures and potential side effects, ensuring a cautious and considered intervention.

The outcomes following corpus callosotomy focus on reducing the severity and impact of generalized seizures rather than eradicating them. By impeding the swift propagation of seizure activity across hemispheres, the procedure aims to enhance overall seizure management and improve the individual's quality of life. Notably, it strives to preserve awareness during seizures, albeit with a reduction in seizure intensity and a potentially improved postictal recovery phase.

However, corpus callosotomy does come with its limitations and potential side effects. It may not address focal seizures originating within specific hemispheres, and there is a possibility of disruptions in certain cognitive functions due to the severed connections impacting interhemispheric communication.

The decision to opt for corpus callosotomy hinges on the severity and type of seizures experienced by the individual, the debilitating impact on daily life, and the potential benefits weighed against the inherent limitations and risks. While not a complete solution, corpus callosotomy presents a significant avenue in the spectrum of surgical interventions, offering hope for improved seizure management and an enhanced quality of life for those grappling with severe seizure disorders

Vagus Nerve Stimulation (VNS)

Vagus Nerve Stimulation (VNS) stands as a pioneering surgical intervention at the forefront of epilepsy management, particularly for those facing uncontrolled seizures despite rigorous medical treatments. In this sophisticated procedure, a small device, reminiscent of a pacemaker, is surgically implanted beneath the skin in the chest, connected to the left vagus nerve in the neck. This intricate setup allows for the delivery of mild electrical pulses to the vagus nerve, strategically modulating neural pathways associated with seizures.

63

The procedure's success lies not only in its implantation but also in the careful calibration of stimulation parameters. Programmed to administer regular electrical pulses at predetermined intervals, the VNS device offers a customizable approach to seizure control. This adaptability extends to patients, who can activate the device using a handheld magnet when sensing the onset of a seizure or experiencing an aura, providing an added layer of control.

The outcomes of VNS are marked by its capacity to significantly reduce seizure frequency and severity, particularly for individuals grappling with refractory epilepsy resistant to conventional medications. Notably, the positive impact of VNS often unfolds gradually over time, necessitating regular follow-ups for fine-tuning and monitoring progress. Beyond its direct antiepileptic effects, individuals commonly report enhancements in mood, alertness, and overall quality of life.

While VNS is generally well-tolerated, considerations include its suitability for individuals who have not achieved satisfactory seizure control through medications alone. The decision to embark on VNS is a collaborative one, involving a comprehensive evaluation by the healthcare team and the individual. Potential side effects, such as hoarseness or tingling sensations during stimulation, are transient and can be addressed through adjustments in the stimulation parameters. VNS is often employed as an adjunctive treatment alongside antiepileptic medications, recognizing the variability in effectiveness among individuals.

In essence, Vagus Nerve Stimulation represents not just a surgical innovation but a dynamic neuromodulatory solution in the complex landscape of epilepsy care. Its tailored approach, adaptability, and positive impact on both seizure control and overall well-being underscore its significance as a transformative option for those navigating the challenges of refractory epilepsy.

Responsive Neurostimulation (RNS)

Responsive Neurostimulation (RNS) represents a pioneering and comprehensive strategy in the realm of epilepsy treatment, particularly for individuals confronting persistent challenges with uncontrolled seizures despite rigorous medical interventions. This advanced therapeutic approach involves a highly sophisticated surgical procedure wherein a responsive neurostimulator device is implanted directly into specific regions of the brain implicated in seizure activity.

The surgical implantation of the RNS device, resembling a small and intricately designed neurostimulator, is a meticulous process that requires precision in targeting the brain areas associated with seizure onset. Equipped with electrodes, this device functions as a vigilant sentinel, continuously monitoring neural activity in real-time. Its unique capability lies in the prompt detection of abnormal electrical patterns indicative of an impending seizure. Once identified, the RNS device delivers precisely calibrated electrical stimulation, strategically modulating the aberrant neural pathways to disrupt the progression of the seizure.

One of the notable strengths of RNS lies in its adaptability. The device can be programmed and fine-tuned non-invasively by healthcare providers based on ongoing monitoring and the individual's specific response. This tailored and personalized approach allows for the optimization of seizure control while minimizing potential side effects, a hallmark feature that sets RNS apart in the landscape of epilepsy interventions.

The outcomes observed with RNS are remarkable, particularly in its efficacy in reducing seizure frequency, especially for individuals grappling with focal epilepsy. Research studies have demonstrated significant improvements in seizure management, with some individuals experiencing a substantial decrease in seizure occurrence over time. Moreover, the continuous monitoring provided by RNS offers valuable insights into the dynamic nature of seizure patterns, facilitating ongoing adjustments and refinements to enhance its therapeutic impact.

Considerations for adopting RNS are multifaceted. Its suitability is often assessed for individuals with focal seizures who have not responded adequately to conventional treatments. The decision to undergo RNS is a collaborative one, involving comprehensive evaluations by the healthcare team and the individual. While RNS is generally well-tolerated, potential side effects are carefully considered, and ongoing monitoring ensures adjustments are made to optimize both efficacy and safety.

Deep Brain Stimulation (DBS)

Deep Brain Stimulation (DBS) stands as a cutting-edge and evolving therapeutic strategy in the expansive landscape of epilepsy management, presenting a ray of hope for individuals grappling with persistent and drug-resistant seizures. At its core, DBS involves the meticulous surgical implantation of a neurostimulator device—resembling a pacemaker—into specific and strategically chosen areas of the brain known to modulate seizure activity.

The intricate DBS procedure unfolds with surgical precision, as electrodes are strategically placed into predetermined brain regions intricately linked to seizure genesis. These electrodes establish a connection to a compact device implanted beneath the skin, usually situated in the chest area.

This device becomes the epicenter for emitting controlled electrical pulses, designed to delicately modulate the abnormal firing patterns of neurons associated with seizures. The ultimate goal is to curtail the frequency and severity of seizures, providing relief to those for whom conventional treatments have proven insufficient.

A standout feature of DBS lies in its adaptability and adjustability. Healthcare providers can remotely fine-tune the stimulation parameters, ensuring a personalized and nuanced approach to treatment. This adaptability allows for the optimization of seizure control while minimizing potential side effects, marking a pivotal aspect of DBS that distinguishes it in the realm of epilepsy interventions.

The observed outcomes associated with DBS showcase significant promise, particularly in reducing seizure frequency, offering a glimmer of hope for individuals navigating the complexities of drug-resistant epilepsy. While research on DBS for epilepsy continues to evolve, clinical studies have highlighted its potential efficacy in improving seizure control and enhancing the overall quality of life for specific individuals.

However, the decision to pursue DBS is a multifaceted process. Typically reserved for individuals contending with drug-resistant focal epilepsy and unresponsive to other interventions, the decision-making journey involves thorough evaluations by healthcare teams and patients alike. The aim is to carefully weigh potential benefits against risks, considering the intricacies of the individual's specific condition and medical history.

Despite being generally well-tolerated, DBS is not without considerations. Potential risks and side effects, including surgical complications, device-related issues, or effects on mood and cognition, necessitate ongoing monitoring and adjustments to optimize the efficacy and safety of the intervention.

In essence, Deep Brain Stimulation emerges as a beacon of progress in the landscape of epilepsy therapeutics. Its adaptive nature, potential efficacy in seizure control, and ongoing advancements position it as a promising frontier in epilepsy care. DBS not only offers hope but also opens up new possibilities for individuals seeking improved seizure management and an enhanced quality of life, marking it as a transformative intervention in the journey against epilepsy.

Hemispherectomy

Hemispherectomy stands as a remarkable and unconventional surgical procedure in the realm of epilepsy treatment, offering a unique solution for individuals confronted with severe and intractable seizures originating from one hemisphere of the brain. This procedure involves the removal, disconnection, or functional isolation of an entire cerebral hemisphere, a bold and intricate intervention designed to disrupt the aberrant neural circuits responsible for recurrent seizures.

The decision to pursue hemispherectomy is typically reserved for individuals with severe epilepsy, often arising from conditions such as Rasmussen's encephalitis, hemimegalencephaly, or other hemispheric pathologies. These conditions may lead to uncontrollable seizures, developmental delays, and other neurological challenges, warranting a comprehensive and individualized approach to treatment.

The surgical process of hemispherectomy requires meticulous planning and execution. Surgeons carefully disconnect or remove the affected hemisphere, aiming to preserve vital structures while effectively isolating the epileptogenic focus. The extent of the procedure varies, with options ranging from anatomic hemispherectomy, where the entire hemisphere is removed, to functional hemispherectomy, preserving the outer cortical layer for cosmetic and structural reasons.

Remarkably, the brain exhibits a remarkable capacity for adaptation following hemispherectomy, especially in young individuals. The remaining hemisphere often takes on functions previously performed by the removed hemisphere, a phenomenon known as neuroplasticity. This adaptability contributes to improved postoperative outcomes, with many individuals experiencing a significant reduction in seizure frequency and, in some cases, substantial improvements in cognitive and developmental outcomes.

Despite its success in mitigating seizures, hemispherectomy is not without consideration. Potential complications include the risk of neurological deficits, visual field impairments, and motor difficulties, which necessitate careful preoperative evaluation and ongoing postoperative rehabilitation and support.

In essence, hemispherectomy represents a bold and effective intervention for individuals facing the debilitating impact of severe epilepsy originating from one cerebral hemisphere. While reserved for select cases, this surgical innovation stands as a testament to the advances in epilepsy treatment, offering a transformative option for those seeking relief from relentless seizures and the associated challenges they bring.

Surgical options for epilepsy require a thorough assessment of each individual's condition, considering factors such as seizure types, brain regions involved, and overall health. While these interventions carry risks, advancements in surgical techniques and ongoing research contribute to improving outcomes and expanding treatment possibilities. Collaboration between healthcare providers and individuals with epilepsy is paramount in making informed decisions and optimizing the potential benefits of surgical interventions.

Holistic Approaches

Holistic approaches to epilepsy management transcend the boundaries of traditional medical interventions, integrating complementary and alternative methods to address the diverse facets of well-being. This comprehensive strategy acknowledges the interconnectedness of physical, mental, and emotional health, providing individuals with epilepsy with a diverse set of tools for managing their condition. Let's delve into a detailed exploration of various complementary and holistic methods integral to this approach:

Mind-Body Techniques

Mind-body techniques stand as integral pillars in the holistic approach to managing epilepsy, recognizing the profound interconnection between mental and physical well-being. These practices empower individuals to cultivate a harmonious relationship between the mind and body, potentially contributing to stress reduction and enhanced emotional resilience.

One key facet of mind-body techniques is mindfulness, a practice that involves cultivating heightened present-moment awareness. Through mindfulness, individuals learn to observe thoughts and sensations without judgment, fostering a sense of calm and reducing the impact of stressors that may act as triggers for seizures. Meditation, a sibling to mindfulness, extends the benefits by offering diverse techniques such as focused attention meditation, loving-kindness meditation, and body scan meditation. These practices equip individuals with tools to enhance mental clarity, emotional balance, and overall well-being.

Yoga and Tai Chi emerge as dynamic mind-body practices that weave physical postures, controlled breathing, and meditation into a holistic tapestry. In yoga, various styles such as Hatha, Kundalini, or Restorative Yoga cater to individual preferences, promoting flexibility, strength, and relaxation. Tai Chi, rooted in traditional Chinese martial arts, engages individuals in slow, flowing movements and focused breathing, fostering balance, coordination, and stress reduction.

Breathwork, exemplified by diaphragmatic breathing and pranayama techniques, becomes a powerful ally in the mind-body journey. Deep, intentional breathing elicits a relaxation response, calming the nervous system and potentially influencing seizure triggers related to emotional stress.

Guided imagery and visualization serve as avenues for mental escape and relaxation. Guided imagery involves creating a mental sanctuary through visualization, offering a refuge from stressors. Visualization techniques extend to envisioning positive outcomes and affirmations, harnessing the mind's power to foster a positive mindset and emotional well-being.

Biofeedback, encompassing electromyography (EMG) and electroencephalography (EEG) biofeedback, provides individuals with tools for self-regulation. EMG biofeedback aids in gaining awareness and control over muscle tension, contributing to overall stress reduction. EEG biofeedback, or neurofeedback, explores the potential of training individuals to modify brainwave patterns, with ongoing research examining its role in seizure management.

In summary, mind-body techniques offer versatile tools within the holistic framework of epilepsy management. While not replacements for medical treatments, their integration reflects a commitment to nurturing a balanced mind-body connection. As part of a comprehensive care strategy, these techniques empower individuals to actively participate in their well-being, fostering resilience and providing valuable tools to navigate the challenges of epilepsy.

Dietary Interventions

Dietary interventions emerge as a crucial component in the holistic management of epilepsy, recognizing the intricate interplay between nutrition, seizure control, and overall health. These interventions provide individuals with epilepsy an expansive avenue to complement conventional medical treatments, fostering a comprehensive strategy to enhance their well-being.

The Ketogenic Diet stands out as a therapeutic cornerstone, involving a meticulously calculated high-fat, low-carbohydrate, and moderate-protein regimen. This specialized dietary approach induces a metabolic state known as ketosis, where the body predominantly utilizes fats for energy. Research indicates its efficacy, particularly in reducing seizures, making it a focal point for individuals, especially children, with specific epilepsy types. However, the implementation of the ketogenic diet necessitates not only commitment but also ongoing monitoring to uphold nutritional equilibrium.

Beyond dietary modifications, the integration of Nutritional Supplements assumes a critical role in addressing potential nutrient deficiencies associated with epilepsy medications or specific dietary restrictions. Guided by healthcare professionals, individuals explore supplements such as vitamin D, calcium, and omega-3 fatty acids, ensuring a comprehensive approach to optimize overall health and well-being.

Herbal and Nutritional Therapies extend the spectrum of dietary interventions, offering a complementary dimension to epilepsy management. Individuals may explore the potential calming effects of herbs like lavender, lemon balm, or skullcap. Simultaneously, engaging in Nutritional Counseling with registered dietitians ensures a holistic and well-balanced eating plan, strategically supporting overall health and nutritional requirements.

Dietary Counseling, a collaborative venture with registered dietitians or nutritionists, tailors dietary plans to address specific needs. This personalized approach considers individual factors such as age, lifestyle, and potential dietary triggers, optimizing the efficacy of dietary strategies. Regular consultations provide ongoing support and adaptation to individual responses.

Individuals may opt for Exploring Elimination Diets to discern and manage potential food triggers for seizures. These systematic approaches involve the deliberate removal and subsequent reintroduction of specific foods or food groups, allowing for observation of any corresponding changes in seizure activity. However, undertaking such interventions mandates professional guidance to prevent nutritional imbalances and deficiencies.

The exploration of Fasting and Intermittent Fasting introduces a dynamic aspect to epilepsy management. Studied for their potential impact on seizure control, these practices are undertaken under the guidance of healthcare professionals, emphasizing the imperative need to maintain nutritional equilibrium during such dietary modifications.

In summation, dietary interventions weave a rich tapestry in the holistic landscape of epilepsy management. While not intended as standalone replacements for medical treatments, these interventions provide a complementary and expansive dimension to the overall strategy. The collaborative engagement with healthcare professionals ensures a tailored, dynamic, and responsive approach, empowering individuals to navigate the complexities of epilepsy with a holistic emphasis on well-being, nutrition, and seizure control.

Stress Management and Counseling

In the holistic realm of epilepsy care, stress management, and counseling emerge as pivotal components, acknowledging the profound impact of emotional well-being on overall health. Individuals navigating the complexities of epilepsy often encounter heightened stress levels, which can potentially act as triggers for seizures. As such, the integration of effective stress management techniques and counseling strategies becomes instrumental in optimizing seizure control and enhancing the overall quality of life.

Expanding therapeutic options, counseling and psychotherapy offer individuals diverse avenues to address the emotional intricacies associated with epilepsy. Cognitive-behavioral therapy (CBT), a cornerstone in this domain, assists individuals in identifying and addressing stressors while fostering the development of coping mechanisms. Beyond CBT, psychodynamic therapy and acceptance and commitment therapy (ACT) provide alternative paths, allowing for tailored approaches based on individual needs and preferences.

Diving into the specifics of therapeutic interventions, biofeedback methods emerge as a nuanced approach to enhance self-regulation, holding promise for stress reduction and seizure management.

Techniques such as electromyography (EMG) and electroencephalography (EEG) biofeedback provide real-time information about physiological processes. EMG biofeedback focuses on muscle activity, aiding in achieving relaxation and reducing muscle tension, while EEG biofeedback offers insights into brainwave patterns, potentially contributing to stress reduction and enhanced seizure control.

In essence, the amalgamation of stress management and counseling not only addresses the emotional dimensions of living with epilepsy but also fosters a holistic approach to well-being. By empowering individuals with effective coping strategies and providing insights into self-regulation through biofeedback, this comprehensive approach seeks to enhance emotional resilience, reduce stress, and contribute to more effective seizure management. Recognizing the individualized nature of the journey with epilepsy, these integrated strategies underscore the importance of tailored care to nurture emotional well-being.

Acupuncture and Acupressure

In the ever-evolving landscape of epilepsy care, traditional healing practices, notably acupuncture and acupressure, are garnering increased attention for their holistic approaches, offering alternative avenues of support for individuals navigating the multifaceted challenges associated with epilepsy.

Originating from ancient Chinese medicine, acupuncture involves the precise insertion of thin needles into specific points on the body. While research continues to explore its direct impact on seizure control, acupuncture has found a niche as a complementary therapy addressing broader aspects of well-being. Beyond potential contributions to seizure management, acupuncture is embraced for its reported efficacy in reducing stress, alleviating anxiety, and enhancing overall mental and physical equilibrium. Its holistic approach aligns with the comprehensive care philosophy, acknowledging the interconnectedness of various facets of health.

Closely akin to acupuncture, acupressure offers a non-invasive alternative by applying pressure to specific points on the body. This gentle technique aims to stimulate the flow of energy, known as "qi," along the body's meridians. Within the realm of epilepsy care, acupressure is considered not only for its potential in stress alleviation but also for its broader impact on promoting relaxation and fostering a more balanced state of being. The gentle yet intentional touch of acupressure aligns with the holistic philosophy of addressing not just the symptoms but the overall well-being of the individual.

The potential benefits of acupuncture and acupressure transcend their role in seizure control. Advocates propose that these ancient practices influence the body's energy flow, contributing to a sense of calmness and overall well-being. While not positioned as standalone treatments for epilepsy, their inclusion in a comprehensive care plan reflects an understanding of the interconnected nature of physical, mental, and emotional health. The holistic benefits of these practices resonate with the broader narrative in healthcare that emphasizes a patient-centric approach to enhance overall quality of life.

One of the notable strengths of acupuncture and acupressure lies in their adaptability to individual needs. Practitioners customize sessions based on a person's unique health profile, taking into account factors such as overall health, stress levels, and specific concerns related to epilepsy. This individualized approach aligns seamlessly with the contemporary trend in healthcare, emphasizing personalized, patient-centered care as a means to enhance overall well-being.

In conclusion, acupuncture and acupressure emerge not just as historical practices but as dynamic elements in the modern epilepsy care paradigm. While ongoing research seeks to further elucidate their direct impact on seizures, their recognized holistic benefits and adaptability underscore their potential contributions to a comprehensive and individualized approach to care. Individuals considering the incorporation of these practices are encouraged to engage in open communication with their healthcare team to ensure safe, coordinated, and patient-centric care.

While these holistic approaches offer additional support, they are not standalone substitutes for medical treatments. The integration of complementary approaches into the overall epilepsy management plan requires ongoing communication and coordination with healthcare professionals. This collaborative and detailed integration exemplifies a holistic approach that empowers individuals to engage actively in their well-being and navigate the complex landscape of epilepsy with a diverse set of tools.

Chapter Three: Navigating Life with Epilepsy

This chapter initiates an in-depth exploration of the multifaceted experiences individuals undergo while living with epilepsy. From subtle nuances to overt challenges, we delve into the intricacies that epilepsy introduces into everyday life. Educational pursuits and professional aspirations intersect with the impact of epilepsy, shaping the landscape of learning and work. Relationships take center stage, offering insights into how epilepsy influences family dynamics and friendships. Within these narratives, we uncover strategies that foster independence and autonomy, providing a roadmap to maintain personal agency while gracefully managing the intricacies of life with epilepsy.

Daily Challenges

Living with epilepsy entails confronting a myriad of nuanced challenges that permeate various aspects of daily life, demanding adaptive strategies and resilience. At the forefront is the capricious nature of seizures, disrupting routine activities and instilling a constant need for vigilance. The emotional strain intensifies as individuals grapple with the fear of experiencing seizures in public or during critical tasks, impacting emotional well-being and daily decision-making.

Navigating the intricate landscape of medication management represents a significant hurdle. While strict adherence to antiepileptic drugs is paramount for seizure control, individuals often contend with potential side effects that necessitate ongoing adjustments. The intersection of epilepsy with educational pursuits and professional aspirations complicates the journey, with discrimination in educational settings or the workplace acting as formidable barriers to academic and career success.

Transportation emerges as a considerable concern, particularly for those facing driving restrictions due to seizures. The reliance on public transportation or the assistance of others may curtail independence, shaping daily routines and lifestyle choices. Cognitive challenges, encompassing epilepsy-related fatigue, memory issues, and cognitive difficulties, further underscore the multifaceted nature of daily functioning.

Social challenges permeate the fabric of relationships as individuals confront societal attitudes and misconceptions about epilepsy. Navigating family dynamics, romantic relationships, and friendships necessitates continuous open communication and understanding to counteract the fear of judgment or rejection. The profound impact on mental health becomes increasingly apparent, with anxiety and depression often accompanying the persistent uncertainty of managing a chronic condition.

Lifestyle adjustments become a recurrent theme, with individuals meticulously considering triggers such as sleep patterns, stress levels, or specific stimuli. Dietary considerations, including the potential impact of certain foods on seizure control, contribute additional layers to the intricacies of daily management. Financial challenges may emerge due to healthcare costs, influencing employment opportunities and overall financial well-being.

In confronting these multifaceted challenges, the indispensable role of a robust support system becomes evident. Family, friends, and healthcare providers are pivotal in providing emotional support, understanding, and practical assistance. The cultivation of coping mechanisms, including mindfulness practices and stress-reduction techniques, becomes paramount for individuals to fortify their resilience amidst the ongoing complexities.

In essence, the daily challenges of living with epilepsy demand a comprehensive, individualized approach to care. Recognizing the unique circumstances and strengths of each person navigating this intricate terrain is essential for fostering a holistic and supportive environment.

Educational and Employment Aspects

The influence of epilepsy on education and employment extends beyond medical considerations, weaving into the very fabric of individuals' aspirations and daily pursuits. In the realm of education, students with epilepsy often encounter a complex interplay of academic challenges and social dynamics. Seizures, particularly if frequent or unpredictable, may disrupt classroom activities, leading to missed lessons and potential gaps in understanding. This disruption can impact educational progress, requiring tailored support and accommodations to ensure an inclusive learning environment.

Beyond the classroom, the stigma surrounding epilepsy can manifest in the form of discrimination or misunderstanding from peers and educators. Misconceptions about the condition may contribute to social isolation, affecting not only academic performance but also the overall well-being of the student. Open communication, awareness campaigns, and support networks are crucial to fostering a positive educational experience for individuals with epilepsy.

Transitioning to the professional sphere, epilepsy can introduce unique challenges in securing and maintaining employment. Employers may harbor misconceptions about the condition, leading to discriminatory practices. Job tasks that involve heightened stress levels or require a high degree of safety consciousness may pose additional challenges. Disclosures about epilepsy in the workplace can be complex, with individuals weighing the benefits of openness against potential biases.

Balancing the demands of work life with the need for regular medical appointments and the potential side effects of medications is an ongoing consideration. Employment opportunities may be curtailed due to driving restrictions or safety concerns in certain industries. Navigating workplace accommodations, such as flexible schedules or modified tasks, becomes essential for fostering a supportive and inclusive work environment.

Moreover, epilepsy's impact on cognitive function may present challenges in tasks that require sustained attention, memory recall, or rapid decision-making. These cognitive considerations can influence job performance and career advancement. Education and advocacy efforts are vital to dispelling myths, promoting workplace inclusivity, and ensuring that individuals with epilepsy have equal opportunities for professional growth.

In conclusion, the educational and employment aspects of living with epilepsy are multifaceted, encompassing academic progress, social dynamics, and professional pursuits. Addressing these aspects necessitates not only medical management but also a broader societal shift towards awareness, understanding, and inclusive practices in educational institutions and workplaces. Empowering individuals with epilepsy to navigate these spheres with confidence and providing the necessary support systems are crucial steps toward fostering an inclusive society.

Relationship Dynamics

The repercussions of epilepsy ripple through the intricate fabric of familial and friendship relationships, introducing both challenges and opportunities for growth. In the familial realm, the diagnosis initiates a cascade of emotions and adjustments. Concerns about the safety and well-being of the individual during seizures prompt family members to navigate a complex emotional landscape.

Anxiety, coupled with a sense of helplessness, underscores the need for transparent and open communication within the family unit. This communication is essential not only for understanding the medical aspects of epilepsy but also for collectively devising strategies for seizure management and emotional support.

The dynamics within the family undergo adaptation as roles are redefined to accommodate the needs of the individual with epilepsy. Siblings, in particular, may grapple with a mix of protective instincts and concerns, influencing the nature of their relationships. Parental roles may evolve to strike a delicate balance between providing necessary support and encouraging the independence of the individual with epilepsy.

In romantic relationships, the impact of epilepsy introduces distinctive challenges that require thoughtful navigation. Honest communication about the condition lays the groundwork for trust and understanding. The unpredictable nature of seizures necessitates partners to collaboratively navigate feelings of fear or uncertainty, fostering resilience and mutual support. Building awareness about epilepsy within the relationship is crucial for dispelling misconceptions and fortifying the emotional bonds between partners.

Within the realm of friendships, the influence of epilepsy is felt in nuanced ways. Misunderstandings about the condition may lead to social isolation or strained relationships. Friends may grapple with the uncertainty of how to provide support or harbor unfounded fears about witnessing a seizure. Educating and raising awareness within friend circles are pivotal for sustaining healthy relationships. Fostering open dialogue and providing resources on epilepsy contribute to the creation of a supportive and understanding network of friends.

Furthermore, the emotional toll of living with epilepsy can reverberate through an individual's mental health, potentially impacting their relationships. Feelings of isolation, anxiety, or depression may strain connections with loved ones. Prioritizing mental health becomes a shared responsibility, prompting both the individual and their support network to seek professional guidance when needed.

In essence, the dynamics of relationships in the context of epilepsy demand continuous understanding, nuanced communication, and a shared commitment to support. Educational initiatives and awareness-building within family and friend circles become integral to cultivating an environment where individuals with epilepsy feel not only accepted and understood but also supported in their relationships. By navigating these complexities together, families and friends can play a pivotal role in contributing to the holistic well-being of those living with epilepsy.

Independence and Autonomy

The pursuit of independence and autonomy in the face of epilepsy unveils a multifaceted journey that demands a meticulous and expansive approach to address the myriad challenges inherent in this complex condition. At its heart, this journey recognizes that fostering and preserving independence is intricately linked to effectively managing the dynamic nuances of epilepsy.

One of the pivotal facets of this quest is the realm of transportation independence, a domain often thrust into focus due to driving restrictions stemming from seizures. As individuals embark on navigating this transition, the exploration of alternative transportation modes becomes not just a practical necessity but a cornerstone in maintaining a sense of agency and freedom. Establishing robust transportation networks or embracing adaptive solutions is imperative to mitigate the impact on mobility, ensuring a sustained sense of independence.

Interwoven with the considerations of transportation are the spheres of employment and education, integral components in the pursuit of autonomy. Open and transparent communication about epilepsy within workplace and educational settings is paramount to establishing the necessary accommodations. Crafting strategies that align with personal career or educational goals while taking into account the potential impacts of seizures becomes a fundamental aspect. The exploration of remote work or flexible scheduling emerges as a strategic endeavor to not only preserve but also enhance professional autonomy.

Central to the comprehensive strategy for independence is the domain of healthcare management. It serves as the bedrock, demanding proactive engagement in one's health journey. Consistent adherence to prescribed medications, regular medical check-ups, and an in-depth understanding of personal seizure triggers emerge as critical elements. Empowering individuals with the knowledge and tools to actively participate in their healthcare decisions not only fosters a sense of control but also enhances their capacity to navigate the multifaceted landscape of epilepsy.

Lifestyle adjustments surface as pivotal contributors to the delicate balance between independence and seizure management. The meticulous development of routines that prioritize not only the medical aspects but also holistic well-being – encompassing adequate sleep, stress reduction techniques, and a commitment to a healthy lifestyle – becomes a robust and interconnected strategy. These adjustments not only contribute to seizure prevention but empower individuals to proactively engage in their daily lives, fostering a profound sense of self-determination.

Within the expansive canvas of social interactions, cultivating a supportive network emerges as an instrumental and ongoing endeavor for maintaining independence. Educating family, friends, and colleagues about epilepsy becomes a catalyst for building a safety net during times of need. Open and continuous conversations about the condition are not merely informative but serve as the foundation for fostering an environment where individuals feel not only understood but actively supported in their relentless pursuit of autonomy.

Harnessing the power of technological advancements unfolds as a significant ally in the journey toward independence. Wearable devices or mobile applications that meticulously track seizures, medication schedules, or stress levels empower individuals to actively manage their health. Embracing assistive technologies, such as alert systems or smart home devices, becomes not just a convenience but an integral part of a comprehensive strategy, contributing to a heightened sense of autonomy.

In essence, the pursuit of independence and autonomy for individuals grappling with epilepsy demands an intricate, detailed, and expansive approach. It necessitates proactive measures across various dimensions of life, encompassing transportation, employment, healthcare, lifestyle, and social interactions. By equipping individuals with epilepsy with a holistic framework of comprehensive strategies and fostering robust support systems, it becomes not just a journey but a profound odyssey toward navigating the delicate balance between autonomy and effective seizure management.

Chapter 4: Emotional and Mental Well-being

In the chapter on Emotional and Mental Well-being, the focus centers on the intricate interplay between epilepsy and individuals' emotional landscapes. It explores coping mechanisms, offering essential strategies to navigate the emotional intricacies of living with epilepsy. This section delves into the potential impact on mental health, highlighting the multifaceted relationship between epilepsy and emotional well-being. Emphasizing the pivotal role of support networks and the significance of seeking professional help, it lays the groundwork for fostering mental resilience. Addressing pervasive stigma, the chapter provides insights and methods to counter societal misconceptions associated with this neurological condition, promoting a more informed and empathetic understanding.

Coping Mechanisms

Living with epilepsy necessitates a holistic approach that extends beyond medical management to encompass the intricate emotional challenges associated with this condition. Here, we delve into an expansive array of coping mechanisms, each meticulously tailored to empower individuals in navigating the multifaceted aspects of their unique journey:

Education and Understanding: Comprehensive knowledge forms the cornerstone of effective coping. Beyond mere awareness, individuals are encouraged to immerse themselves in educational resources, actively participate in support groups, and engage in open dialogues with healthcare professionals. This depth of understanding not only demystifies epilepsy but also equips individuals to proactively manage the accompanying anxiety and uncertainty.

Mindfulness and Stress Management: Cultivating mindfulness practices, such as mindfulness meditation and guided imagery, becomes pivotal in reducing stress and fostering emotional well-being. These practices extend beyond mere relaxation techniques; they serve as powerful tools in recognizing stress as a potential trigger for seizures, contributing not only to emotional resilience but also to optimized seizure control.

Cognitive Behavioral Therapy (CBT): As a structured therapeutic approach, CBT aids individuals in identifying and modifying negative thought patterns. The goal is to equip them with practical skills to effectively manage stress, anxiety, and depression. By fostering emotional resilience and cultivating a positive mindset, CBT becomes an integral component of coping with the challenges presented by epilepsy.

Journaling and Self-Reflection: The practice of journaling is encouraged as a tangible outlet for emotional expression. By documenting emotions, seizure patterns, and triggers, individuals engage in a process of self-reflection. This not only aids in identifying patterns but also becomes a valuable tool during discussions with healthcare providers, fostering a deeper understanding of their journey with epilepsy.

Peer Support and Counseling: The significance of connecting with others who share similar experiences through peer support groups cannot be overstated. This creates a sense of community, allowing for the sharing of feelings, insights, and mutual encouragement. Simultaneously, professional counseling, specifically tailored to address the unique emotional challenges associated with epilepsy, provides invaluable guidance and coping strategies.

Emotional Regulation Techniques: Practical techniques for emotional regulation, including deep breathing exercises, progressive muscle relaxation, and biofeedback, serve as empowering tools. These techniques not only aid in managing intense emotions and stress but also become essential components of the emotional resilience toolkit, fostering an enduring sense of balance.

Creating a Supportive Environment: Fostering an understanding and supportive environment involves an ongoing process of educating friends, family, and colleagues about epilepsy. This not only reduces feelings of isolation but also encourages open communication, creating a supportive safety net during challenging times.

Healthy Lifestyle Practices: Emphasizing healthy lifestyle practices contributes significantly to overall well-being. Regular exercise, balanced nutrition, adequate sleep, and limitations on alcohol and caffeine intake impact physical health and may concurrently reduce seizure frequency while enhancing emotional resilience.

Art Therapy and Creative Expression: Encouraging engagement in creative outlets like art, music, or writing serves as a therapeutic avenue for emotional expression. Creative pursuits become means to process emotions, reduce stress, and enhance emotional well-being.

Exploration of Holistic Practices: Under professional guidance, exploring complementary therapies such as acupuncture, aromatherapy, or herbal remedies becomes an additional dimension of emotional balance. These holistic approaches, when integrated with traditional treatments, contribute to emotional well-being and overall wellness.

In essence, the integration of these diverse and detailed coping mechanisms creates a robust and personalized toolkit. Empowered by these tools, individuals with epilepsy can actively manage their emotions, fostering resilience and navigating the emotional landscape of their journey with increased confidence, adaptability, and a holistic approach.

Mental Health and Epilepsy

Living with epilepsy immerses individuals in a profound psychological journey, where the complexities of the condition intertwine with the intricacies of mental well-being. This section delves deeper into the multifaceted ways in which epilepsy can impact mental health, recognizing the nuances that shape the emotional landscape:

Psychological Complexity: Epilepsy introduces a psychological landscape marked by diversity. Beyond anxiety and depression, individuals grapple with a spectrum of emotions, including fear, frustration, and uncertainty. Understanding this intricate emotional tapestry is vital for tailoring interventions that address the nuanced aspects of mental health.

Social Stigma and Isolation: The stigmatization associated with epilepsy casts a shadow on mental well-being. Discrimination and societal misconceptions contribute to a pervasive sense of isolation.

Overcoming this stigma requires not only societal shifts but also individual empowerment to navigate social relationships with resilience and self-assurance.

Quality of Life Considerations: Epilepsy's chronic nature reverberates through various dimensions of life, influencing overall quality. The interplay between physical restrictions, safety concerns, and potential limitations in personal and professional pursuits becomes a psychological terrain that requires careful navigation, impacting the mental well-being of those on this journey.

Coping with Uncertainty: The perpetual uncertainty introduced by the unpredictable nature of seizures is a central psychological challenge. Beyond the fear of seizures themselves, the anticipation and uncertainty surrounding when seizures might occur contribute to heightened stress levels. Developing effective coping strategies for managing this uncertainty becomes a crucial aspect of mental health management.

Cognitive Impact and Emotional Resilience: Cognitive challenges, such as memory issues and difficulties with concentration, add layers of complexity to the emotional landscape. Frustration and concerns about cognitive decline become emotional hurdles. Building emotional resilience becomes imperative, emphasizing not just the cognitive impacts but also the adaptive strategies that empower individuals to navigate these challenges.

Interpersonal Dynamics and Relationship Strain: Epilepsy's influence extends beyond the individual to interpersonal relationships. The emotional strain stemming from concerns about the well-being of the person with epilepsy and potential impacts on relationships becomes a psychological challenge. Nurturing healthy relationships requires not just individual coping mechanisms but also open communication and mutual understanding.

Medication Side Effects and Emotional Well-being: While antiepileptic medications are indispensable for seizure control, their side effects can impact emotional well-being. Mood swings, changes in cognition, or alterations in energy levels may occur, necessitating a nuanced approach to medication management that considers both seizure control and emotional health.

Holistic Approaches and Proactive Mental Health Care: Recognizing the interplay between epilepsy and mental health underscores the importance of proactive and holistic interventions. Integrating mental health support into epilepsy care involves not just counseling but also comprehensive psychoeducation. Holistic approaches, including mindfulness practices, stress management techniques, and peer support, create a robust framework that empowers individuals to navigate the emotional complexities of epilepsy with resilience and enhanced well-being.

Support Networks

In the intricate tapestry of life with epilepsy, the role of support networks takes on multifaceted dimensions, offering a comprehensive framework that extends beyond mere emotional solace. This detailed exploration delves into the nuanced layers of support, recognizing their distinct contributions to the well-being of individuals navigating the challenges of epilepsy:

Family and Friends: Immediate family and close friends form the foundational layer of support. Beyond emotional encouragement, educating them about epilepsy becomes a profound mechanism for fostering a supportive environment. This educational aspect extends beyond seizure first aid to encompass an understanding of the emotional impact of epilepsy, contributing to a holistic approach to support.

Peer Support Groups: Peer support groups, whether conducted in person or through virtual platforms, serve as crucibles of shared experience. These forums provide not only a space for individuals with epilepsy to exchange coping strategies but also a haven where the nuances of their journeys are deeply understood. In-depth discussions on managing the emotional toll, dealing with societal attitudes, and navigating relationships foster a sense of community.

Educational and Workplace Support: Beyond the immediate circle, educational and workplace environments play pivotal roles in an individual's life. Establishing understanding and support in these settings is paramount. Educators and employers equipped with knowledge about epilepsy contribute to creating inclusive environments that accommodate the unique needs of individuals with epilepsy. This inclusivity transcends the academic and professional realms, shaping a broader support structure.

Professional Healthcare Providers: The collaboration with healthcare providers transcends the clinical realm, encompassing a holistic approach to care. Regular communication ensures not only optimal management of the physical aspects of epilepsy but also addresses the psychological and emotional dimensions. In-depth discussions on treatment plans, potential side effects, and strategies for navigating daily challenges contribute to a nuanced understanding of the individual's experience.

Psychological Support: Mental health, intricately intertwined with epilepsy, necessitates specialized support. Psychologists, counselors, and psychiatrists become integral components of the support network, offering tailored interventions for managing the emotional impact of epilepsy. Exploring coping mechanisms, addressing stigma-related concerns, and providing a safe space for expression contribute to a holistic approach to mental well-being.

Community Organizations and Advocacy Groups: Engaging with community organizations and advocacy groups dedicated to epilepsy broadens the support horizon. These groups not only offer a wealth of resources and educational materials but also spearhead awareness campaigns and advocate for the rights and well-being of individuals with epilepsy. Becoming actively involved in these organizations not only expands the support network but also empowers individuals to effect positive change.

Online Resources and Forums: The digital landscape, replete with forums, blogs, and reputable websites dedicated to epilepsy, emerges as a dynamic support arena. Online platforms provide continuous access to information, facilitating a virtual support network that transcends geographical boundaries. Interactive discussions, expert insights, and shared experiences contribute to a sense of belonging and connection.

Emergency Response Training: Empowering the support network with practical skills enhances safety. Training family and friends in seizure first aid, and emergency response strategies, and creating a comprehensive emergency plan ensure a proactive and secure environment. This layer of support not only addresses immediate safety concerns but also cultivates a sense of preparedness and confidence.

Crisis Intervention and Helplines: In acknowledgment of potential crises, awareness of and access to helplines and crisis intervention services becomes crucial. A robust support network is not only cognizant of these resources but actively encourages individuals with epilepsy to seek immediate assistance during challenging times. This layer of support becomes a lifeline during critical moments.

Empowering the Individual: A support network that goes beyond external assistance to empower the individual is pivotal. Encouraging self-advocacy, fostering independence, and actively involving the individual in decision-making contribute to a support system that recognizes their agency. This empowerment extends to the cultivation of skills for effective self-management and resilience-building.

In conclusion, the depth and effectiveness of a support network for individuals with epilepsy lie in its ability to recognize and address the nuanced aspects of their journey. By acknowledging the diverse layers of support, we not only create a safety net but also foster an environment where individuals can navigate the complexities of epilepsy with resilience, empowerment, and a profound sense of community.

Dealing with Stigma

Navigating life with epilepsy entails confronting societal stigma, an intricate challenge rooted in historical misconceptions and a pervasive lack of understanding. This detailed exploration delves into the nuanced landscape of stigma associated with epilepsy, unraveling its multifaceted dimensions and providing comprehensive strategies for individuals to overcome these pervasive challenges.

Understanding Epilepsy-Related Stigma: The roots of stigma surrounding epilepsy run deep, stemming from historical misconceptions, ingrained cultural beliefs, and a prevailing lack of awareness. Individuals often find themselves grappling with prejudiced attitudes, discrimination, and social isolation, creating formidable barriers to education, employment, and meaningful social interactions.

Educational Initiatives: Education emerges as a powerful counterforce against stigma. Tailored awareness campaigns aimed at schools, workplaces, and communities prove instrumental in dispelling myths and offering accurate information about epilepsy. Inclusive educational materials, dynamic presentations, and facilitated discussions collectively contribute to fostering an environment where epilepsy is understood as a medical condition rather than a source of unwarranted fear.

Media Representation and Advocacy: The media's role in shaping public perceptions is pivotal. Advocacy efforts must strategically focus on encouraging accurate and empathetic portrayals of epilepsy across various media outlets. Personal narratives, thought-provoking documentaries, and insightful interviews play a transformative role in humanizing the condition, challenging stereotypes, and actively contributing to reshaping societal attitudes.

Community Engagement: Building robust connections within communities stands as a vital strategy for breaking down entrenched barriers. Open dialogues about epilepsy, thoughtfully curated community events, and the active involvement of individuals with epilepsy in diverse activities collectively serve to normalize the condition. This proactive engagement not only fosters inclusivity but also acts as a potent force in diminishing the fear associated with the unknown.

Legal Protections and Anti-Discrimination Policies: The implementation and reinforcement of legal protections against discrimination represent a cornerstone in the battle against stigma. Advocacy for robust anti-discrimination policies in workplaces and public spaces becomes a crucial mechanism to ensure that individuals with epilepsy enjoy the same rights and opportunities as their peers. These legal frameworks act not only as safeguards but also as powerful deterrents against discriminatory practices.

Peer Support and Mentorship Programs: Creating purposeful spaces for individuals with epilepsy to connect and support each other stands as a cornerstone in fostering a sense of community. Peer support groups and mentorship programs offer valuable avenues for sharing experiences, developing effective coping strategies, and providing advice on navigating the intricate landscape of societal challenges. This collective support becomes a catalyst, empowering individuals to confront and triumph over the prevailing stigma.

Counseling and Mental Health Support: Dealing with the pervasive impact of stigma on mental health underscores the need for targeted support services. Offering counseling services tailored to address the emotional fallout of stigma becomes a crucial element. Mental health professionals equipped with coping strategies, resilience-building techniques, and a safe space for expression play a pivotal role in aiding individuals in navigating the complex emotional landscape.

Public Advocacy and Celebrities: Engaging influential public figures and celebrities to advocate for epilepsy awareness represents a significant and impactful strategy. Their influence has the potential to draw attention to the unique challenges faced by individuals with epilepsy, challenge ingrained stereotypes, and encourage positive societal change. Celebrities openly discussing their experiences contribute substantially to normalizing the condition.

Empowerment Through Education: Providing individuals with epilepsy the tools and knowledge to educate others takes center stage in empowerment endeavors. Comprehensive training programs, encompassing self-advocacy skills, effective communication strategies, and nuanced ways to educate peers, collectively contribute to breaking down barriers. Empowered individuals, armed with knowledge, become potent advocates for change within their immediate circles.

Cultural Sensitivity Training: Acknowledging and addressing cultural beliefs and practices contributing to stigma becomes a critical aspect of the comprehensive strategy. Cultural sensitivity training tailored for healthcare professionals, educators, and community leaders serves as a bridge, fostering understanding and promoting inclusivity and respect for diverse perspectives.

In conclusion, the battle against and triumph over epilepsy-related stigma requires a concerted, multifaceted effort from individuals, communities, and society at large. Through strategic educational initiatives, targeted media representation, community engagement, robust legal frameworks, peer support programs, mental health services, public advocacy, and cultural sensitivity training, it is possible to dismantle the entrenched barriers perpetuating stigma. In doing so, a world can be fostered where individuals with epilepsy are not only embraced for their resilience but celebrated for their valuable contributions to society.

Chapter Five: Lifestyle Modifications

In the chapter on Lifestyle Modifications, we delve into essential aspects that play a pivotal role in managing epilepsy, offering a holistic approach to well-being. Exploring the intersection of diet and nutrition, we uncover the influence these factors have on epilepsy management. The significance of physical activity and its impact on seizures is discussed, emphasizing the importance of exercise for overall health. Addressing the intricate relationship between sleep patterns and seizures, we shed light on the crucial role of proper sleep in epilepsy management. Additionally, stress management takes center stage as we unravel strategies for stress reduction and its vital role in promoting optimal health for individuals navigating life with epilepsy.

Diet and Nutrition

Diet and nutrition play multifaceted roles in the comprehensive management of epilepsy, intricately woven into the fabric of overall health and the nuanced dynamics of seizures. This detailed exploration delves into various dimensions of the relationship between diet, nutrition, and epilepsy control, offering a thorough understanding of how dietary choices can exert profound effects on seizure frequency and severity.

Balancing Macronutrients for Stability

Balancing macronutrients for stability is a fundamental aspect of dietary management, particularly in the context of promoting health and managing conditions such as epilepsy. The term "macronutrients" refers to the three primary components of the diet: carbohydrates, proteins, and fats. Achieving a harmonious balance among these macronutrients is essential for maintaining overall well-being and, in the case of epilepsy, for potentially influencing seizure control.

Carbohydrates are a primary source of energy for the body. They are converted into glucose, serving as the energy source for diverse bodily functions, including the functioning of the brain. In the context of epilepsy, the impact of carbohydrates on blood glucose levels is of particular significance. Managing carbohydrate intake involves understanding the concept of the glycemic index, which measures how quickly a carbohydrate-containing food raises blood glucose levels. Balancing complex carbohydrates, which have a slower impact on blood sugar, with fiber-rich choices can contribute to more stable energy levels and potentially influence seizure control.

Proteins are crucial for building and repairing tissues, including muscles, organs, and enzymes. In the context of balancing macronutrients, ensuring an adequate intake of protein is essential for maintaining overall health. Protein-rich foods can contribute to satiety, helping individuals feel fuller for longer periods. This can be particularly relevant for those managing epilepsy, as stable blood sugar levels and sustained energy can play a role in seizure management.

Dietary fats are diverse and can be classified into saturated fats, unsaturated fats, and trans fats. Fats are essential for various bodily functions, including the absorption of fat-soluble vitamins and the production of hormones. In recent years, the ketogenic diet, which is high in fats and low in carbohydrates, has gained attention for its potential impact on epilepsy. The diet aims to induce a state of ketosis, where the body relies on ketones for energy instead of glucose. Research suggests that this metabolic shift may have positive effects on seizure control in some individuals.

Achieving a balanced intake of carbohydrates, proteins, and fats involves mindful food choices and portion control. This can be facilitated by focusing on whole, nutrient-dense foods, such as fruits, vegetables, lean proteins, and healthy fats. Paying attention to individual dietary needs, considering factors like age, activity level, and health status, is crucial for tailoring macronutrient intake.

In the realm of epilepsy management, discussions about macronutrients often intersect with dietary approaches like the ketogenic diet. While research is ongoing, some individuals with epilepsy may explore dietary modifications, guided by healthcare professionals, to assess their impact on seizure control.

In essence, balancing macronutrients for stability is about adopting a holistic and individualized approach to dietary choices. By understanding the roles of carbohydrates, proteins, and fats in the body and tailoring their intake, individuals can contribute to overall health and potentially influence factors relevant to epilepsy management.

Ketogenic Diet and Seizure Control

The ketogenic diet, a high-fat, low-carbohydrate eating plan, has gained attention for its potential impact on seizure control, particularly in individuals with epilepsy. The diet is designed to induce a state of ketosis, where the body shifts from using glucose as its primary energy source to relying on ketones, produced from fats, for energy. This metabolic shift is believed to have anticonvulsant effects, influencing the frequency and intensity of seizures in some individuals.

The ketogenic diet's influence on seizure control is rooted in its ability to alter the metabolic environment of the brain. When carbohydrates are restricted, the body produces ketones, which become an alternative fuel source for the brain. This shift in energy metabolism is thought to reduce hyperexcitability in the brain, a factor associated with seizures.

112

Research indicates that the ketogenic diet can be effective in reducing seizures, especially in certain types of epilepsy that may not respond well to traditional medications. It has shown particular promise in children with epilepsy, leading to some becoming seizure-free or experiencing a significant reduction in seizure frequency. The diet's impact on seizure control varies among individuals, and its effectiveness may depend on factors such as specific epilepsy syndrome, age, and adherence to the diet.

The ketogenic diet is a specialized, medically supervised dietary intervention. It typically involves a carefully calculated ratio of fats to carbohydrates and proteins. There are different variations of the ketogenic diet, including the classic ketogenic diet, the modified Atkins diet, and the low glycemic index treatment. These variations allow for some flexibility in food choices while maintaining the key principles of low-carbohydrate, high-fat intake.

While the ketogenic diet has demonstrated efficacy, it is not without challenges. Adherence can be demanding, as the diet requires strict macronutrient ratios. Potential side effects, such as nutrient deficiencies and gastrointestinal issues, may also arise. Regular monitoring by healthcare professionals is essential to address these concerns and optimize the diet's benefits while minimizing risks.

The ketogenic diet is typically considered when other treatment options, such as antiepileptic medications, have not provided sufficient seizure control. It is often implemented under the guidance of a multidisciplinary healthcare team, including neurologists, dietitians, and other specialists. The decision to incorporate the ketogenic diet into epilepsy management is individualized, considering factors such as the individual's overall health, lifestyle, and preferences.

In conclusion, the ketogenic diet's potential for influencing seizure control has positioned it as a valuable adjunctive therapy for certain individuals with epilepsy. Its implementation requires careful consideration and supervision to ensure safety and optimize its impact on seizure management. While not a one-size-fits-all solution, the ketogenic diet exemplifies the evolving landscape of personalized approaches to epilepsy care.

Micronutrients and Neurological Health

Micronutrients, encompassing a spectrum of vital vitamins and minerals, are instrumental in supporting neurological function, neurotransmitter synthesis, and the overall well-being of the brain. The B-vitamin complex, comprising thiamine, pyridoxine, and cobalamin, stands as a cornerstone for energy metabolism and neurotransmitter synthesis, sourced from nutrient-rich foods such as whole grains, leafy greens, eggs, and dairy products.

Vitamin D, pivotal for calcium absorption, bone health, and immune function, finds its sources in sunlight exposure, fatty fish, and fortified dairy products. Moving to omega-3 fatty acids, prevalent in fatty fish, flaxseeds, chia seeds, and walnuts, these essential compounds contribute not only to brain structure but also play a role in neurotransmitter function and exhibit anti-inflammatory properties, potentially influencing seizure control.

Magnesium, derived from nuts, seeds, leafy greens, and whole grains, emerges as a key mineral essential for neurotransmission and with potential modulatory effects on neuronal excitability. Zinc, found in meat, dairy, legumes, and nuts, contributes to neurotransmitter synthesis and supports immune function. Meanwhile, antioxidant vitamins C and E, sourced from citrus fruits, berries, nuts, seeds, and vegetable oils, play a pivotal role in combating oxidative stress, providing neuroprotection against seizures.

In navigating the landscape of micronutrient intake in epilepsy management, considerations extend to individual variability, potential medication interactions, dietary diversity, and the judicious use of supplementation when necessary. A varied and balanced diet, enriched with a spectrum of colorful fruits, vegetables, whole grains, and lean proteins, forms the bedrock of ensuring optimal micronutrient intake.

This holistic approach to micronutrient support necessitates addressing specific deficiencies, promoting overall dietary quality, and tailoring interventions to individualized needs. Recognizing the intricate interconnectedness of micronutrients and neurological health not only complements other facets of epilepsy management but also contributes to an enriched understanding that fosters enhanced overall well-being.

Potential Triggers and Dietary Considerations

Identifying potential triggers involves a thorough examination of individual responses to certain foods or dietary elements. Some individuals may find that specific food additives, preservatives, or stimulants present in processed foods act as triggers, influencing seizure activity. Caffeine, a known stimulant, can also impact seizure thresholds. Notably, alcohol, when consumed excessively, has the potential to elevate the risk of seizures. Furthermore, exploring potential food allergies or intolerances is crucial, highlighting the importance of allergy testing and consultation with healthcare professionals for a comprehensive understanding.

On the positive side, strategic dietary considerations can be integral to epilepsy management. The ketogenic diet, characterized by high fat and low carbohydrates, has demonstrated efficacy in reducing seizures, especially in pediatric cases. This diet induces a metabolic state that produces ketones, offering an alternative energy source. Another dietary approach involves emphasizing a low glycemic index (GI), focusing on foods that stabilize blood sugar levels.

Nutrient-dense choices, such as fruits, vegetables, whole grains, and lean proteins, contribute not only to overall health but also potentially to seizure control.

Maintaining proper hydration is a fundamental consideration, as dehydration can influence seizure thresholds. Individuals with epilepsy are encouraged to uphold adequate fluid intake. It is crucial to recognize that dietary strategies should be personalized, considering factors like age, general health, lifestyle, and medication interactions. Collaboration with healthcare professionals, particularly dietitians, is invaluable for tailoring dietary recommendations to individual needs.

In conclusion, this exhaustive exploration illuminates the pivotal and multifaceted role of diet and nutrition in epilepsy management. By comprehending the delicate balance of macronutrients, unraveling the intricacies of specialized diets like the Ketogenic Diet, acknowledging the significance of micronutrients, addressing potential dietary triggers, and embracing personalized nutrition plans, individuals with epilepsy gain the knowledge and agency to navigate toward optimal seizure control through informed, nuanced, and empowered dietary choices.

Exercise and Physical Health

Regular physical activity is not only integral for overall health but holds particular relevance for individuals managing epilepsy. The intricate interplay between exercise and epilepsy involves a myriad of positive effects that extend beyond the physical realm. While the direct impact of exercise on seizure frequency can be variable among individuals, the holistic benefits contribute significantly to an overall sense of well-being.

First and foremost, exercise is a cornerstone of cardiovascular health, promoting a robust circulatory system that nourishes the brain with oxygen and nutrients. The neurovascular coupling, the intricate relationship between neuronal activity and blood flow, is crucial for optimal brain function. By enhancing this coupling, exercise potentially contributes to the maintenance of healthy neuronal networks.

Beyond the physiological aspects, exercise is a potent mood regulator. The release of endorphins during physical activity, often referred to as the "runner's high," is associated with improved mood and reduced stress. Given that stress is recognized as a potential trigger for seizures in some individuals, incorporating regular exercise can positively impact stress levels and potentially influence seizure thresholds.

Moreover, exercise has been linked to neuroprotective mechanisms, fostering the growth and maintenance of neurons. Neurotrophic factors, substances that support the survival, development, and function of neurons, are released during exercise. This neuroplasticity, or the brain's ability to adapt and reorganize, is crucial in the context of epilepsy, where maintaining optimal brain health is paramount.

In addition to its impact on mood and neuroprotection, exercise is intertwined with sleep quality. Establishing a consistent sleep pattern is crucial for individuals with epilepsy, as sleep disruptions can potentially trigger seizures. Regular physical activity contributes to better sleep hygiene, promoting a healthy sleep-wake cycle and potentially reducing seizure susceptibility associated with sleep disturbances.

Despite these myriad benefits, safety considerations are paramount for individuals with epilepsy engaging in physical activity. Healthcare providers play a crucial role in assessing individual health status, determining appropriate exercise intensity and type, and offering personalized recommendations. Factors such as seizure type, overall health, and any comorbidities should inform the development of tailored exercise plans.

A diversified approach to exercise, encompassing aerobic activities, strength training, and flexibility exercises, can provide comprehensive health benefits. While individualized exercise recommendations are crucial, fostering a supportive and inclusive environment for individuals with epilepsy to engage in physical activities is equally essential. The holistic benefits of exercise underscore its role as a valuable component in the comprehensive management of epilepsy.

Sleep and Epilepsy

Understanding the symbiotic relationship between epilepsy and sleep unveils a vast spectrum of influences that permeate both seizure occurrence and the overall health landscape of individuals coping with epilepsy. The intricate dance between sleep patterns and seizures is nuanced; any deviations in sleep quality or disruptions in the sleep-wake cycle can significantly impact seizure occurrences. Sleep deprivation or irregular sleep not only diminishes the overall quality of sleep but can also diminish the seizure threshold, rendering individuals more susceptible to experiencing seizures.

Conversely, seizures themselves can wreak havoc on the natural sleep cycle. Nocturnal seizures, disrupt the normal course of sleep, fragment sleep cycles, and lead to daytime drowsiness, fatigue, and compromised cognitive and physical functioning during waking hours. This complex interplay highlights the bidirectional relationship between epilepsy and sleep, each profoundly affecting the other.

Moreover, the body's internal clock, known as circadian rhythms, holds sway over the timing of seizures. Certain forms of epilepsy exhibit circadian patterns, making seizures more likely at specific times of day or night. Unraveling these patterns is crucial for tailoring treatment strategies to maximize their effectiveness and minimize disruption to daily life.

Establishing sound sleep hygiene practices is fundamental for individuals managing epilepsy. Consistent sleep routines, conducive sleep environments, and minimizing stimulants before bedtime are vital steps in promoting healthy sleep patterns. The potential impact of a stable and supportive sleep routine extends beyond merely improving sleep quality; it might also influence seizure frequency and enhance overall well-being.

Additionally, monitoring and diagnosing sleep disorders form a critical part of comprehensive epilepsy care. Conditions such as sleep apnea, insomnia, or restless legs syndrome can exacerbate epilepsy symptoms and profoundly affect overall health. Addressing these comorbidities becomes integral to a holistic approach to epilepsy management.

Responses to sleep interventions are highly individualized, calling for personalized approaches considering seizure type, lifestyle, and specific health needs. Close collaboration with healthcare providers, including specialists in sleep medicine, serves to elucidate an individual's unique sleep patterns, paving the way for effective management of any underlying sleep disorders.

By recognizing and navigating the intricate relationship between sleep and epilepsy, individuals gain empowerment to proactively manage their condition. Tailoring interventions to individual needs holds the promise of potentially reducing seizure frequency, improving overall health, and significantly enhancing the quality of life for those navigating life with epilepsy.

Stress Management

Navigating the intricate relationship between stress and epilepsy is crucial for comprehensive management and overall well-being. Stress, whether physical or emotional, is recognized as a common trigger for seizures in individuals with epilepsy. The bidirectional influence of stress and epilepsy creates a complex interplay, necessitating thoughtful strategies for stress reduction.

Strategies for stress management in the context of epilepsy encompass a multifaceted approach. Understanding individual stressors is the first step, allowing for tailored interventions. Lifestyle modifications, such as adopting regular exercise routines, engaging in relaxation techniques (including deep breathing and meditation), and fostering a consistent sleep schedule, contribute significantly to stress reduction.

Cognitive-behavioral therapy (CBT) is an evidence-based therapeutic approach that proves valuable in addressing stress-related triggers. CBT assists individuals in identifying and reframing negative thought patterns, building coping mechanisms, and enhancing resilience. Psychoeducation is another essential component, empowering individuals with epilepsy to recognize stressors and implement effective stress reduction strategies.

Mindfulness-based stress reduction (MBSR) programs offer valuable tools for cultivating mindfulness and increasing awareness of the present moment. Through mindfulness practices, individuals can develop a heightened sense of self-awareness, enabling them to manage stress more effectively and mitigate its impact on epilepsy.

Social support networks play a pivotal role in stress management. Open communication with friends, family, and healthcare providers fosters a supportive environment where individuals can share their concerns and receive encouragement. Support groups, both in-person and online, provide platforms for connecting with others facing similar challenges, creating a sense of community and shared understanding.

Maintaining a healthy work-life balance is integral to stress reduction. Strategies may involve setting realistic goals, prioritizing tasks, and establishing boundaries to prevent burnout. Professional support, including counseling or workplace accommodations, can contribute to a more supportive and conducive work environment.

Regular self-assessment is essential in stress management for individuals with epilepsy. Recognizing signs of stress and proactively addressing them helps prevent the escalation of stress-related triggers. Developing personalized stress reduction plans, in collaboration with healthcare providers, ensures that interventions align with individual needs and are integrated into the overall epilepsy management strategy.

Ultimately, stress management in the context of epilepsy is a dynamic process that evolves. Embracing a holistic approach, integrating various stress reduction strategies, and acknowledging the unique aspects of individual experiences contribute to more effective stress management. By navigating stress proactively, individuals with epilepsy can enhance their overall quality of life and optimize seizure control.

Chapter Six: Looking Towards the Future

This chapter serves as a portal into the ever-evolving landscape of epilepsy care. From delving into current and future advancements in research to uncovering the transformative role of technology in epilepsy management, this chapter encapsulates the dynamic trajectory of the field. It extends its focus to unveil strategies and innovations dedicated to elevating the quality of life for individuals navigating epilepsy, promising a more holistic approach to care. Amidst these discussions, the chapter interweaves narratives of resilience and hope, showcasing the indomitable spirit within the epilepsy community. As we embark on this journey into the future, these insights pave the way for a more promising and compassionate era in epilepsy care.

Advancements in Research

Epilepsy research stands at the forefront of a transformative era characterized by multifaceted advancements that promise to redefine our understanding and management of this neurological condition. The intricate landscape of genetic research in epilepsy is unfolding, providing unprecedented insights into the role of specific genes in predisposition and susceptibility. This genetic knowledge is steering the trajectory towards precision medicine, where interventions are tailored based on an individual's unique genetic makeup, fostering a new era of targeted and personalized treatment strategies.

The realm of neuroimaging contributes significantly to this evolving narrative. The advent of advanced technologies, such as functional magnetic resonance imaging (fMRI) and sophisticated electroencephalogram (EEG) analyses, enables researchers to delve into the intricacies of brain activity during seizures. This heightened granularity in understanding facilitates precise localization of abnormal neural activity, paving the way for nuanced and individualized treatment approaches.

The confluence of technology and epilepsy management has brought forth groundbreaking innovations, fundamentally altering the patient experience. Wearable devices and mobile applications, designed for real-time seizure monitoring, empower individuals by providing valuable insights into their seizure patterns. This data-driven paradigm fosters a collaborative approach between patients and healthcare providers, facilitating informed decision-making and more personalized treatment plans.

The future trajectory of epilepsy research is poised for further revolutionary developments. Explorations into gene therapies, aiming to address the root causes of epilepsy at the genetic level, hold immense promise for transformative treatments.

Neuromodulation techniques, which involve modulating neural circuits to control seizures, represent another frontier in the pursuit of more effective therapeutic interventions.

The integration of artificial intelligence (AI) and machine learning stands as a compelling paradigm in epilepsy research. These technologies, armed with the capacity to analyze vast datasets, can discern intricate patterns in epilepsy dynamics and treatment responses. This data-driven approach holds the potential to unlock personalized treatment strategies, optimize therapeutic outcomes, and reshape the landscape of epilepsy care.

Furthermore, international collaboration and active patient engagement are becoming integral components of the research narrative. The collective efforts of researchers, clinicians, and individuals affected by epilepsy are amplifying the impact of these advancements. By merging scientific rigor, technological innovation, and a patient-centric ethos, the future of epilepsy research appears to be a beacon of hope, promising enhanced treatment efficacy, improved quality of life, and increased resilience for those navigating the complexities of epilepsy.

Improving Quality of Life

Improving the quality of life for individuals with epilepsy involves a multifaceted approach that encompasses various strategies and innovative interventions. The goal is to address not only the medical aspects of epilepsy but also the broader impact it has on daily life, mental well-being, and social interactions.

Educational Programs: Comprehensive educational programs play a pivotal role in disseminating accurate information about epilepsy and reducing societal stigma. These programs, tailored for schools, workplaces, and communities, contribute to a more informed and empathetic environment. Education empowers individuals and fosters understanding, reducing the fear associated with epilepsy.

Holistic Healthcare Approach: In addition to neurologists, a holistic healthcare approach involves incorporating mental health professionals, counselors, and specialists. This ensures that the physical and psychological aspects of epilepsy are addressed, promoting overall well-being. Collaborative care teams facilitate a more holistic understanding of the challenges faced by individuals.

Psychosocial Support Services: Psychosocial support services, including counseling and support groups, offer individuals with epilepsy a platform to share experiences, coping mechanisms, and emotional challenges. This fosters a supportive network and addresses the emotional toll of living with epilepsy. Emotional well-being is a crucial aspect of overall quality of life.

Employment Support and Vocational Programs: Employment support and vocational programs empower individuals with epilepsy to pursue meaningful work. These initiatives aim to reduce stigma, break down employment barriers, and enhance financial independence. Meaningful employment contributes significantly to an individual's sense of purpose and self-worth.

Assistive Technologies: Leveraging assistive technologies, such as seizure detection devices and smart home technologies, significantly enhances safety and quality of life. These technologies provide real-time monitoring and support, contributing to a sense of security and independence. They empower individuals to live more confidently.

Creating an Inclusive Society: Creating an inclusive society involves initiatives that improve physical accessibility and raise awareness to reduce societal stigma. Advocating for policies that protect the rights and opportunities of individuals with epilepsy is crucial for fostering inclusivity. Inclusion contributes to a sense of belonging and acceptance.

Personalized Therapeutic Interventions: Personalized therapeutic interventions, including medication adjustments, cognitive-behavioral therapy, and regular assessments, ensure that treatment plans align with the evolving needs of each individual. This personalized approach optimizes the effectiveness of interventions, addressing individual challenges.

Recreational and Leisure Activities: Access to inclusive recreational and leisure activities tailored to individual preferences promotes social integration and overall well-being. Participating in sports, arts, and cultural activities contributes to a fulfilling and balanced lifestyle. Leisure activities offer avenues for relaxation and enjoyment.

Seizure Management Plans: Developing individualized seizure management plans involves identifying triggers, implementing lifestyle modifications, and establishing effective communication with healthcare providers. This empowers individuals to actively manage their condition and regain a sense of control. Understanding and managing seizures are integral aspects of epilepsy care.

Advocacy for Policy Changes: Advocacy for policy changes at a systemic level is vital for creating an environment that supports the quality of life for individuals with epilepsy. This includes pushing for anti-discrimination laws, educational accommodations, and workplace policies that safeguard the rights and dignity of those with epilepsy. Policy changes contribute to systemic improvements in societal attitudes and structures.

Stories of Hope and Resilience

Sarah's Journey to Empowerment

Sarah's odyssey toward empowerment commenced during the formative years of adolescence when an epilepsy diagnosis cast shadows of social isolation and self-esteem struggles. The pivotal juncture in her narrative, however, unfolds as a collective endeavor rather than a solitary conquest. Recognizing the intricate layers of her emotional challenges, Sarah immersed herself in therapeutic counseling, seeking solace and understanding. Her trajectory toward empowerment gained momentum as she actively sought and became an integral part of epilepsy support groups—a community offering shared experiences and empathetic bonds.

The narrative acquires depth as Sarah delves into public speaking training, a deliberate choice aimed at overcoming the pervasive fear of judgment that often accompanies epilepsy. Emerging from the cocoon of silence, she embarked on a mission to share her story with local schools and communities. Her engagements served as platforms for fostering profound understanding and dispelling pervasive myths surrounding epilepsy. Through eloquent articulation, Sarah became an advocate for awareness, transforming her journey into a beacon of resilience and education.

Sarah's resilience stands as a profound testament to the transformative power inherent in self-advocacy and community support. Beyond the personal triumph over isolation, her narrative echoes the broader impact of collective understanding and the profound ripple effects that emanate from courageous storytelling. The richness of her journey lies not just in the conquering of personal demons but in the shared illumination she brings to others navigating similar paths. In Sarah's story, empowerment transcends the individual, embracing the collective spirit of empathy, education, and resilience within the epilepsy community.

Jason's Artistic Triumph

Jason's artistic triumph unfolds as a compelling narrative woven into the intricate tapestry of his emotional journey with epilepsy. Far more than a visual endeavor, his art transcends traditional boundaries, transforming into a tactile and emotional experience for those who encounter it. The genesis of Jason's creative process involves a profound commitment to understanding the neurological nuances of epilepsy, creating a unique intersection between the realms of science and art.

In his quest for authenticity, Jason embarks on meticulous research, delving into the intricacies of the brain's response to epilepsy. This dedication serves as a foundation for his artistic expression, allowing him to portray not just the physical manifestations but also the emotional landscapes of living with epilepsy. Each brushstroke becomes a conduit for translating the internal struggles and triumphs onto canvas, providing viewers with a visceral connection to the human experience.

Jason's impact extends beyond the canvas as he actively engages with the public through gallery exhibitions and collaborations with neuroscientists. These collaborations aim to bridge the gap between scientific understanding and artistic interpretation, fostering a deeper appreciation for the complexities of epilepsy. By merging the subjective realm of emotions with objective insights from neuroscience, Jason's work becomes a vehicle for empathy, education, and destigmatization.

Through his art, Jason invites viewers into the intimate realm of epilepsy, offering a perspective that transcends clinical explanations. The emotional resonance of his creations serves not only as a testament to personal resilience but also as a catalyst for societal empathy and understanding. Jason's artistic triumph stands as a poignant example of the transformative power of creativity in shaping perceptions and fostering dialogue around the multifaceted experiences of individuals living with epilepsy.

A Family's Resilience

The narrative of the Thompson family's resilience unfolds as a testament to their unwavering commitment to not only support their son, Ethan but also to address the broader imperative of fostering community understanding. In a remarkable display of proactive engagement, the Thompsons initiated a transformative project—an endeavor to establish a local support group. This ambitious undertaking necessitated collaboration with healthcare professionals, community leaders, and educators, showcasing the family's determination to create a comprehensive support network.

The heart of the Thompsons' initiative lies in the development of an inclusive community that transcends traditional familial bonds. The establishment of workshops, awareness campaigns, and mentorship programs became instrumental in creating a resilient network capable of offering a lifeline to families navigating the complex landscape of pediatric epilepsy. Through these efforts, the Thompsons aimed not only to provide a source of support for their son but also to extend a supportive hand to other families facing similar challenges.

The workshops hosted by the Thompsons served as knowledge-sharing platforms, equipping community members with essential information about pediatric epilepsy, its management, and the psychosocial aspects associated with the condition. Simultaneously, awareness campaigns sought to destigmatize epilepsy, challenging misconceptions and fostering a more compassionate understanding within the broader community.

The mentorship programs established by the Thompsons added a personal touch to their community-building efforts. Families confronted with the challenges of pediatric epilepsy found solace and guidance through connections with those who had navigated similar journeys. The mentorship structure facilitated a peer-to-peer support system, enriching the community's collective resilience by drawing strength from shared experiences.

Through their multifaceted initiatives, the Thompsons exemplify a holistic approach to resilience—one that extends beyond the familial unit to embrace the community at large. Their story becomes a beacon of hope, illustrating the transformative potential of collective action, education, and support in fostering understanding and resilience within the intricate tapestry of pediatric epilepsy.

Navigating the Workplace

Maya's triumph in the workplace stands as a beacon of pioneering inclusivity, showcasing a narrative of resilience, advocacy, and transformative change. Her journey toward success within the professional realm involved a strategic and collaborative approach, beginning with close collaboration with the human resources department. Maya recognized the importance of creating an environment that not only accommodated her needs as an individual with epilepsy but also paved the way for a more inclusive workplace culture.

Education emerged as a cornerstone of Maya's advocacy efforts. Recognizing the power of awareness in dismantling stereotypes and fostering understanding, Maya took on the role of an educator within her workplace. She conducted informative sessions, workshops, and discussions aimed at enlightening her colleagues about epilepsy – its nuances, challenges, and strategies to create a supportive and empathetic work environment.

In addition to education, Maya spearheaded the introduction of workplace wellness programs specifically designed to accommodate the diverse needs of employees, including those with epilepsy. These initiatives not only catered to the physical and mental well-being of the entire workforce but also served as a testament to Maya's commitment to creating a workplace that prioritizes inclusivity and values the unique contributions of each individual.

Maya's visibility as an advocate for inclusivity was pivotal in challenging pre-existing notions and fostering a corporate culture that embraced diversity. Her courage in sharing her journey with epilepsy helped break down barriers and create an atmosphere where open dialogue and understanding could flourish. This cultural shift went beyond Maya's individual experiences, influencing the broader corporate landscape by setting a precedent for the inclusivity and accommodation of individuals with epilepsy.

Maya's story serves as an inspirational case study, illustrating the transformative potential of corporate environments when they actively embrace diversity, educate their workforce, and institute policies and programs that champion inclusivity. Her journey exemplifies how individuals with epilepsy can not only navigate the workplace successfully but also act as catalysts for positive change, shaping corporate cultures that prioritize empathy, understanding, and support.

These detailed narratives collectively highlight the diverse ways in which individuals within the epilepsy community navigate challenges, advocate for change, and find sources of strength and hope. Each story contributes to a mosaic of resilience, fostering a sense of community and inspiring others on their unique journeys with epilepsy.

Conclusion

As we draw the final pages of this comprehensive exploration into the vast landscape of epilepsy, it is essential to pause and reflect on the myriad insights and perspectives that have unfolded throughout this journey. The chapters have unraveled the complexities of diagnosis, treatment options, lifestyle modifications, and the profound impact of epilepsy on various facets of life. In this recap, we stand at the intersection of knowledge and empowerment.

For those navigating the intricate pathways of epilepsy, it's crucial to recognize the strength within. Living with epilepsy is a unique journey, and each individual's experience is as varied and nuanced as the condition itself. As we reflect on the diverse narratives shared within these pages, it becomes evident that resilience, support systems, and a proactive approach can transform challenges into opportunities for growth.

To those living with epilepsy, I extend words of encouragement and empowerment. Your journey is a testament to your strength and tenacity. Embrace the uniqueness of your story, for it contributes to the diverse tapestry of the epilepsy community. Remember that you are not alone. Seek support from your loved ones, engage with support groups, and embrace the wealth of resources available.

Taking proactive steps in managing your condition is an act of self-empowerment. Stay informed about the latest advancements, collaborate with healthcare professionals, and actively participate in your treatment plan. Advocate for awareness within your community, dispelling myths and fostering understanding. Your voice is a powerful instrument in dismantling stigma and shaping a more compassionate world.

As we conclude this chapter, I want to convey a personal message of hope and solidarity within the epilepsy community. Each person touched by epilepsy is part of a global network connected by shared experiences. In the face of challenges, find solace in the collective strength and resilience that unites us. Let us move forward with hope, compassion, and a shared commitment to building a world where individuals with epilepsy are embraced for their unique contributions.

In closing, this book is not just an exploration of epilepsy; it is a testament to the human spirit's capacity to overcome, adapt, and thrive. May the insights gained here be a source of empowerment, and may the words resonate as a reminder that, together, we can create a future where epilepsy is understood, stigma is dismantled, and every individual can live a life of fulfillment and dignity.

Dear Valued Reader,

We trust you've found inspiration and insight within the pages of "Thriving Beyond Seizures." Your engagement with this narrative is vital, and we would be honored to hear your reflections. If the book has resonated with you, we kindly invite you to share your thoughts on platforms such as Amazon, Goodreads, or any other review site of your choice.

Your review not only aids us in refining our work but also serves as a guiding light for others navigating similar paths. Your candid feedback is a crucial part of our collective effort to foster understanding, resilience, and hope within the epilepsy community.

We genuinely appreciate your time, consideration, and the significant role you play in this literary journey. Your reviews go beyond words; they become beacons of support for those seeking empowerment beyond seizures. Thank you for being an essential part of this shared commitment.

With heartfelt thanks and warm regards,

Kari Wallis,

Author of Thriving Beyond Seizures.

Made in the USA
Las Vegas, NV
09 December 2023

82331734R00079